MW01488804

Uveitis

A Colour Manual of
Diagnosis and Treatment

Uveitis

A Colour Manual of Diagnosis and Treatment

Jack J. Kanski, MD, FRCS

Consultant Surgeon,
Prince Charles Eye Unit,
King Edward VII Hospital,
Windsor

Butterworths
London   Boston   Durban   Singapore
Sydney   Toronto   Wellington

First published 1987

© Butterworth & Co. (Publishers) Ltd, 1987

British Library Cataloguing in Publication Data

Kanski, Jack J.
   Uveitis : a colour manual of diagnosis
   and treatment.
   1. Uveitis
   I. Title
   617.7'2   RE351
   ISBN 0-407-01640-6

Library of Congress Cataloguing in Publication Data

Kanski, Jack J.
   Uveitis : a colour manual of diagnosis and
treatment.

   Includes bibliographies and index.
   1. Uveitis.   I. Title. [DNLM: 1. Uveitis- diagnosis.
2. Uveitis-therapy. WW 240 K16u]
   RE351.K3   1987   617.7'.2   86-20797
   ISBN 0-407-01640-6

Photoset by Scribe Design, Gillingham, Kent
Printed by Toppan Printing Company (H.K.) Ltd, Hong Kong

Preface

Uveitis is a fascinating condition which has many diverse causes and systemic associations. Although the last few years have seen great progress in the management of uveitis, many ophthalmologists are still frequently uncertain and frustrated when faced with a new case. The main aim of this book is to provide the general ophthalmologist and trainee with a systematic approach to the diagnosis and management of this relatively common disease. Each uveitis entity is therefore described in terms of its main clinical features, its clinical course and potential complications, management and differential diagnosis. The colour illustrations are intended to help the reader correctly interpret important clinical signs. The last two chapters are devoted to the management of complicated cataract and secondary glaucoma which are the two most important causes of visual morbidity in patients with uveitis. The bibliography is intended to provide the reader with key references from which he can pursue a particular topic in more depth.

I am greatly indebted to Miss F. Kinnear, Dr A. Evans, and Dr N. Strong for reviewing the manuscript and for making many helpful suggestions. I am also grateful to Mr J. McAllister for his help with Chapter 12. Many of the photographs were taken by Miss Daphne Bannister and the artwork is due to the genius of Terry Tarrant.

Jack J. Kanski

Contents

1

Introduction

Definitions

Uveitis

Although by strict definition uveitis is an inflammation of the uveal tract the term is now used to describe many forms of intraocular inflammation which may involve not only the uvea but also adjacent structures.

Endophthalmitis

This is a severe form of intraocular inflammation involving the ocular cavities and their immediate adjacent structures without extension of the inflammatory process beyond the sclera.

Panophthalmitis

This is similar to endophthalmitis except that the inflammatory process also involves the outer ocular coats as well as Tenon's capsule. In very severe cases, the orbital tissues may also be affected.

Vitritis

This is an infiltration of the vitreous cavity by inflammatory cells either due to uveitis or endophthalmitis.

Vasculitis

This is an inflammation of the retinal blood vessels.

Keratic precipitates

These are cellular deposits on the corneal endothelium.

Classifications

Many classifications of uveitis have been proposed, none of which is perfect. The four most useful classifications are:

1 Anatomical.
2 Clinical.
3 Aetiological.
4 Pathological.

Anatomical classification

Classified anatomically, uveitis can be anterior, intermediate, posterior, or diffuse (*see Figure 1.1*).

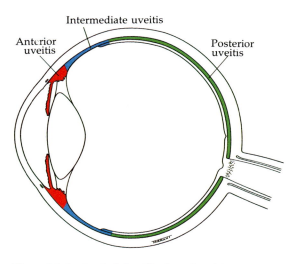

Figure 1.1 Anatomical classification of uveitis

1

Anterior uveitis

Anterior uveitis is subdivided into *iritis* in which the inflammation predominantly affects the iris and *iridocyclitis* in which both the iris and the anterior part of the ciliary body (pars plicata) are equally involved.

Intermediate uveitis

Intermediate uveitis (pars planitis, chronic cyclitis) is characterized by predominant involvement of the posterior part of the ciliary body (pars plana) and the extreme periphery of the retina.

Posterior uveitis

In posterior uveitis the inflammation is located behind the posterior border of the vitreous base. According to the site of primary involvement, posterior uveitis is subdivided into choroiditis, retinitis, chorioretinitis, and retinochoroiditis.

Diffuse or panuveitis

Diffuse or panuveitis is characterized by involvement of the entire uveal tract.

> *Note* Anterior uveitis is the most common type followed by intermediate, posterior, and diffuse.

Clinical classification

Classified according to the mode of onset and duration, uveitis can be acute or chronic.

Acute uveitis

Acute uveitis usually has a sudden symptomatic onset and persists for six weeks or less. If the inflammation recurs following the initial attack it is referred to as acute recurrent.

Chronic uveitis

Chronic uveitis persists for months or years. Its onset is frequently insidious and asymptomatic although occasionally acute or subacute exacerbations of inflammation may occur during the course of a chronic uveitis.

Classified according to severity, uveitis may be *mild* or *severe*.

Aetiological classification

Classified aetiologically, uveitis can be exogenous or endogenous.

Exogenous uveitis

Exogenous uveitis is caused by either external injury to the uvea or by the invasion of micro-organisms or other agents from outside.

Endogenous uveitis

Endogenous uveitis is caused by micro-organisms or other agents from within the patient.

> *Note*
> 1 In many cases of endogenous uveitis the actual cause is unknown.
> 2 The prognosis of exogenous uveitis is usually worse than for endogenous uveitis.
> 3 This book deals mainly with endogenous uveitis.

Classification of endogenous uveitis The six main types of endogenous uveitis are:
1 Secondary to a systemic disease, such as: arthritis, e.g. ankylosing spondylitis; granuloma, e.g. sarcoidosis; chronic infection, e.g. tuberculosis.
2 Parasitic infestations, e.g. toxoplasmosis.
3 Viral infections, e.g. cytomegalovirus.
4 Fungal infections, e.g. candidiasis.
5 Idiopathic specific uveitis entities are a group of unrelated disorders which are not usually associated with any underlying systemic disease but which have special characteristics of their own to warrant a separate description, e.g. pars planitis.
6 Idiopathic non-specific uveitis entities which do not fall into any of the above categories make up about 25% of all cases of uveitis.

Pathological classification

Classified pathologically, uveitis is granulomatous or non-granulomatous. The main clinical differences between the two are summarized in *Table 1.1*.

Table 1.1 Main differences between granulomatous and non-granulomatous uveitis

Feature	Granulomatous	Non-granulomatous
Onset	Insidious	Acute
Course	Long	Short
Anterior segment		
Injection	+	+++
Pain	±	+++
Iris nodules	+++	−
Keratic precipitates	'Mutton fat'	Usually small
Fundus	Nodular lesions	Diffuse involvement

Note Clinically, this distinction is not always useful because some forms of granulomatous uveitis, e.g. sarcoidosis, may present with non-granulomatous features and, occasionally, non-granulomatous inflammation may have granulomatous characteristics.

When describing a patient with uveitis, as many characteristics as possible should be used. For example:

1 A 22-year-old man with lower back pain and a unilateral, acute, severe, non-granulomatous iritis.
2 A 44-year-old female with sarcoidosis and a bilateral, chronic, mild, granulomatous iridocyclitis.
3 A healthy 11-year-old girl with chronic, severe, bilateral, non-granulomatous iridocyclitis.
4 A healthy 15-year-old boy with an acute, unilateral, mild, focal, retinochoroiditis.

Clinical features

Anterior uveitis

Symptoms

The main symptoms of acute anterior uveitis are photophobia, pain, redness, decreased vision and lacrimation. In chronic anterior uveitis, however, the eye may be white and symptoms minimal, even in the presence of severe inflammation.

Signs

Injection In acute anterior uveitis the circumcorneal 'ciliary' injection has a violaceous hue (*Figure 1.2*). The degree of injection should be graded from 0 to +4.

Keratic precipitates The characteristics and distribution of keratic precipitates (KPs) may provide

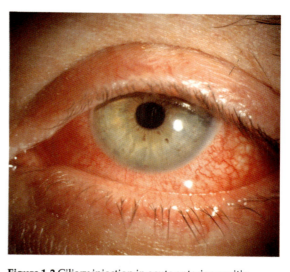

Figure 1.2 Ciliary injection in acute anterior uveitis

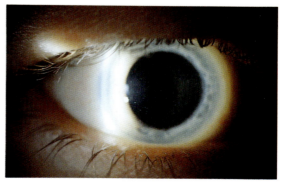

Figure 1.3 Keratic precipitates in Fuchs' uveitis syndrome

clues as to the possible aetiology of the uveitis. The following observations should be made and recorded.

Distribution KPs most commonly form in the mid and inferior zones of the cornea. However, in Fuchs' uveitis syndrome, they are scattered throughout the endothelium (*Figure 1.3*).

Size
1 Endothelial dusting (*Figure 1.4*) by many hundreds of small cells occurs in acute anterior uveitis, as well as during subacute exacerbations of chronic inflammation.
2 Small KPs are characteristic of herpes zoster and Fuchs' uveitis syndrome.
3 Medium KPs occur in most types of acute and chronic anterior uveitis (*Figure 1.5*).

Note The number of KPs should be recorded in the notes because a decrease in KPs usually indicates a favourable response to treatment.

4 Large KPs are usually of the 'mutton fat' variety and have a greasy or waxy appearance (*Figure 1.6*). They are composed of clusters of epithelioid cells and mononuclear macrophages and they typically occur in granulomatous uveitis.

Fresh or old? Fresh KPs tend to be white and round. As they age, they shrink, fade, and become pigmented. Fading 'mutton fat' KPs usually take on a 'ground-glass' (hyalinized) appearance (*Figure 1.7*).

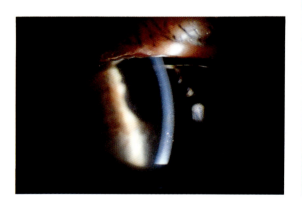

Figure 1.4 Endothelial 'dusting' in acute anterior uveitis

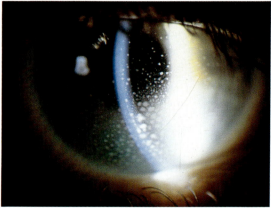

Figure 1.6 'Mutton fat' keratic precipitates

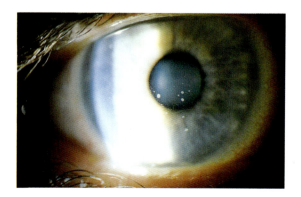

Figure 1.5 Small and medium-size keratic precipitates

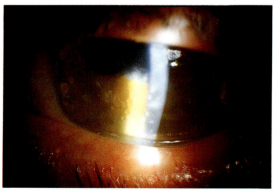

Figure 1.7 Old keratic precipitates

Aqueous cells (Figure 1.8) The cells should be graded according to the number observed in the oblique slit beam. The light intensity and magnification of the slitlamp should be maximal and the beam 3-mm long and 1-mm wide. The cells should be counted and graded from 0 to +4 as shown in *Table 1.2*.

Table 1.2 Grading of aqueous cells

Cells per field	Grade
0	–
1–5	±
5–10	+
10–20	++
20–50	+++
Over 50	++++

Table 1.3 Grading of aqueous flare

Description	Grade
Complete absence	0
Faint—just detectable	+
Moderate—iris details clear	++
Marked—iris details hazy	+++
Intense—fixed coagulated aqueous with considerable fibrin	++++

counting cells. The beam should be passed obliquely to the plane of the iris in order to evaluate the degree of obscuration of iris details. The flare is graded from 0 to +4 as shown in *Table 1.3*.

Note
1 It is important to distinguish inflammatory cells from pigment cells and blood. Inflammatory cells are small, spherical, glistening, and non-pigmented. Macrophages are larger, especially when they have ingested blood or melanin.
2 Always examine the aqueous prior to dilating the pupil because, following pupillary dilatation, a few cells are frequently seen in normal eyes.
3 Cells may be difficult to detect in an eye with a dense flare.

Note A flare is due to leakage of proteins into the aqueous humour through damaged blood vessels and is not necessarily a sign of active uveitis. For this reason, the presence of a flare in the absence of cells is *not* an indication for steroid therapy.

Aqueous flare The grading of flare is performed using the same setting on the slitlamp as for

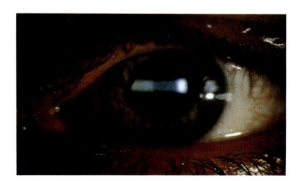

Figure 1.8 Aqueous cells (+4) and dense flare

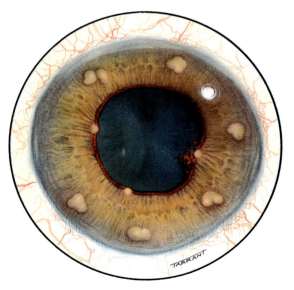

Figure 1.9 Koeppe and Busacca iris nodules in granulomatous anterior uveitis

Iris nodules (Figure 1.9) Koeppe nodules are situated at the pupillary border and are smaller than Busacca nodules which are less common and which are located on the surface of the iris away from the pupil.

> *Note* Although iris nodules are a feature of granulomatous inflammation, Koeppe nodules are sometimes seen in non-granulomatous inflammations such as Fuchs' uveitis syndrome and juvenile chronic iridocyclitis.

Iris atrophy This is an important feature of Fuchs' uveitis syndrome (*Figure 1.10*) and it also occurs in uveitis due to herpes simplex and herpes zoster.

Rubeosis iridis (Figure 1.11) Rubeosis iridis (iris neovascularization) develops in some eyes with chronic anterior uveitis and in Fuchs' uveitis syndrome. In severe cases, a fibrovascular membrane covers the anterior lens surface and occludes the pupil (occlusio pupillae). In a few cases, neovascularization also develops in the chamber angle.

> *Note* Iris neovascularization is frequently associated with a persistent aqueous flare due to the continuous leakage of proteins into the aqueous humour.

Posterior synechiae (Figure 1.12) Posterior synechiae (adhesions between the anterior lens surface and the iris) form with ease during an attack of acute anterior uveitis because the pupil is small. They may also form in eyes with moderate to severe chronic anterior uveitis. Posterior synechiae extending for 360 degrees (seclusio pupillae) prevent the passage of aqueous humour from the posterior to the anterior chamber giving

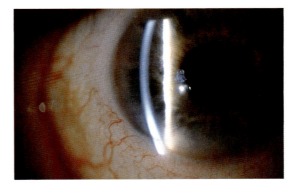

Figure 1.11 Rubeosis iridis in chronic anterior uveitis

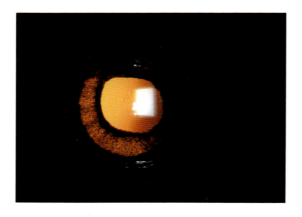

Figure 1.10 Iris atrophy in Fuchs' uveitis syndrome seen on iris transillumination

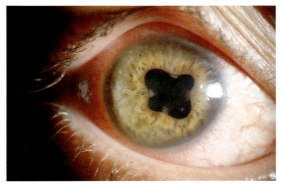

Figure 1.12 Posterior synechiae

rise to a forward bowing of the peripheral iris (iris bombè), which may lead to elevation of intraocular pressure due to secondary closure of the angle by the peripheral iris. In some eyes with chronic anterior uveitis seclusion and occlusion of the pupil occur together.

Note
1 Secondary lens opacities seem to progress more quickly in the presence of posterior synechiae.
2 Pigment on the anterior lens surface is usually indicative of ruptured posterior synechiae.
3 The presence of posterior synechiae excludes the diagnosis of Fuchs' uveitis syndrome in which posterior synechiae never form, even in long-standing cases.

Note Direct and indirect ophthalmoscopy are mandatory in all eyes with anterior uveitis for the following reasons:
1 Some cases of predominantly posterior uveitis, e.g. toxoplasmosis, may cause a 'spill-over' of cells into the aqueous and unless the posterior inflammatory focus is detected the condition may be misdiagnosed as a primary anterior uveitis.
2 Eyes with rhegmatogenous retinal detachments frequently have a mild to moderate secondary anterior uveitis and occasionally posterior synechiae. Unless the fundus is examined the underlying retinal detachment will be missed.
3 Both retinoblastoma and malignant melanoma of the choroid may present with anterior chamber inflammation (masquerade syndrome—*see* later).

Anterior vitreous The cell density in the anterior vitreous (*Figure 1.13*) should be compared with that in the aqueous. In iritis, aqueous cells far exceed the number of vitreous cells, whereas in iridocyclitis the cells are distributed equally between the two compartments.

Posterior segment A careful examination should be performed of the macula for evidence of cystoid macular oedema which is an occasional complication of chronic anterior uveitis and a common complication of intermediate uveitis.

Intermediate uveitis

Symptoms

The presenting symptom is usually floaters, although occasionally the patient presents with impairment of central vision due to chronic cystoid macular oedema.

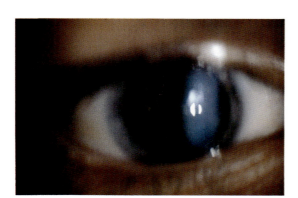

Figure 1.13 Cells in anterior vitreous

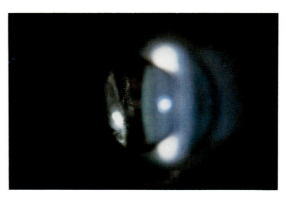

Figure 1.14 'Snowball' vitreous opacities in pars planitis

Signs

Intermediate uveitis is characterized by vitritis with few, if any, cells in the anterior chamber and the absence of a focal inflammatory lesion in the fundus. A mild peripheral retinal periphlebitis occurs in some patients. The hallmark of pars planitis is the presence of a grey-white plaque involving the inferior pars plana which is referred to as 'snowbanking' and small gelatinous exudates in the vitreous called 'snowballs' or 'cotton balls' (*Figure 1.14*).

Posterior uveitis

Symptoms

The two main symptoms of posterior segment inflammation are floaters and impaired vision. A patient with a peripheral inflammatory lesion will complain of seeing floaters and may have only minimal blurring of vision. On the other hand, active choroiditis involving the fovea or papillo-macular bundle will primarily cause loss of central vision and the patient may not notice the presence of floaters.

Signs

Vitreous   Posterior segment inflammation causes vitreous opacities, vitreous flare, and frequently posterior vitreous detachment. The opacities should be classified according to size, shape, and position within the vitreous cavity.

Fine opacities (Figure 1.13) are composed of individual inflammatory cells. In some cases the detached posterior hyaloid face is covered by inflammatory precipitates comparable to KPs.

Coarse opacities are usually the result of severe tissue destruction.

'Snowball' opacities (Figure 1.14) are characteristic of pars planitis, although they may also occur in candidiasis and sarcoidosis.

Stringy opacities (Figure 1.15) are usually caused by alterations in the vitreous gel itself.

Note   The posterior two-thirds of the vitreous are evaluated using a slitlamp and one of the following lenses: (1) Goldmann contact lens, (2) Hruby lens, and (3) a + 90 dioptre aspheric lens (Volk). The latter, which gives the same image as an indirect ophthalmoscope, is best for evaluating vitreoretinal relationships such as posterior vitreous detachment, whereas the Goldmann contact lens is particularly useful for detecting vitreous cells.

Grading of vitreous activity   Grading of vitreous activity is less satisfactory than grading of anterior chamber activity. It can be performed with either the direct or indirect ophthalmoscope.

With direct ophthalmoscope   The old grading system proposed by Kimura, Thygeson and Hogan (1959) is shown in *Table 1.4*.

Table 1.4 Grading of vitreous activity using direct ophthalmoscope

Description	Grade
No opacities	0
Few scattered fine and coarse opacities with a clear view of the fundus	+
Scattered fine and coarse opacities with fundus details somewhat obscured	++
Many opacities with marked blurring of fundus	+++
Dense opacities with no view of fundus	++++

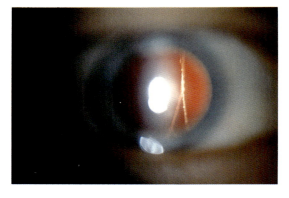

Figure 1.15 Stringy vitreous opacities

Table 1.5 Grading of vitreous activity with indirect ophthalmoscope

Description	Grade
Optic nerve head obscured	++++
Optic nerve head visible but borders blurred	+++
Better visualization of retinal blood vessels	++
Better definition of optic nerve head and retinal blood vessels	+
Blurring of retinal nerve fibre striations	±
Nerve fibre striations well defined	0

With indirect ophthalmoscope The disadvantage of the old grading system is that, in some eyes with active inflammation, vitreous cells and opacities may persist for many months despite the fact that the vitreous haze has resolved and visual acuity has returned to normal. For this reason, Nussenblatt and associates (1985) have proposed that the severity of *vitreous activity* is best assessed by grading the extent of vitreous haze. This is performed with the pupil maximally dilated with the indirect ophthalmoscope beam set at mid-power and a +20 dioptre lens. The clarity of three fundus landmarks are used as criteria: optic nerve head, retinal blood vessels, and normal striations and reflex of the retinal nerve fibres. The haze is then graded as shown in *Table 1.5.*

> *Note* Vitreous clearing first occurs furthest away from the inflammatory focus.

Fundus

Choroiditis (Figure 1.16) is characterized by yellow or greyish patches with reasonably well-demarcated borders. Inactive lesions appear as white well-defined areas of chorioretinal atrophy with pigmented borders. The retinal blood vessels, which may be sheathed, pass over the lesions undisturbed.

Retinitis (Figure 1.17) gives the retina a white cloudy appearance. Because the outline of the inflammatory focus is indistinct, exact demarcation between healthy and inflamed retina may be difficult to discern.

> *Note* Posterior segment inflammation can be focal (*Figure 1.16*), multifocal (*Figure 1.18*), geographical (*Figure 1.19*) and diffuse.

Vasculitis may involve the retinal veins (periphlebitis) or, less commonly, the arterioles (periarteritis). Active periphlebitis is characterized by a fluffy white haziness surrounding the blood

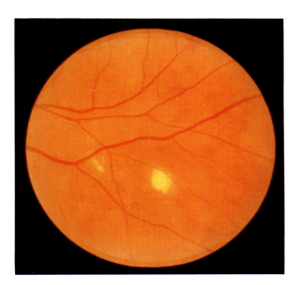

Figure 1.16 Active focal choroiditis (courtesy of Mr A. Shun-Shin)

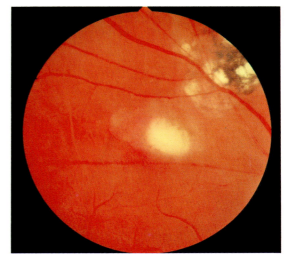

Figure 1.17 Active focal retinochoroiditis

column. Involvement is patchy, with irregular extensions outside the vessel wall. It represents a chronic inflammatory cell infiltrate within and surrounding the vessel wall, which may resolve without sequelae or it may be replaced by venous sclerosis.

Note   Perivascular accumulation of granulomatous tissue in severe periphlebitis gives rise to 'candlewax drippings' or 'candlewax exudates' (Figure 1.20).

Neovascularization   is relatively rare in eyes with posterior segment inflammation, although sarcoidosis may be associated with both peripheral as well as disc new vessels. Because the new vessels are not usually associated with significant areas of capillary closure, they frequently regress once the inflammation is controlled although, on occasion, they may cause vitreous haemorrhage.

Retinal detachment   Exudative retinal detachment is the hallmark of Harada's disease. Rhegmatogenous and/or tractional retinal detachment is a common complication of acute retinal necrosis, and it occasionally occurs in eyes with severe toxoplasmosis and pars planitis.

Optic nerve head   findings include papillitis (from contiguous or distant inflammatory foci), oedema (from hypotony), granuloma (sarcoidosis), and optic atrophy (secondary to retinal damage).

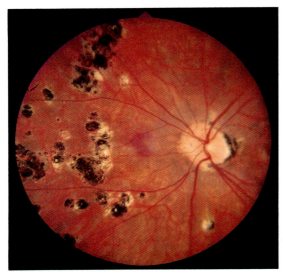

Figure 1.18 Old multifocal retinochoroiditis

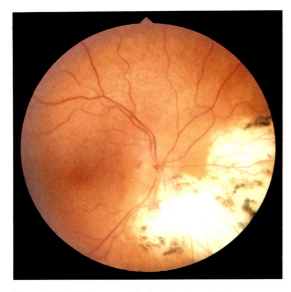

Figure 1.19 Old geographical retinochoroiditis

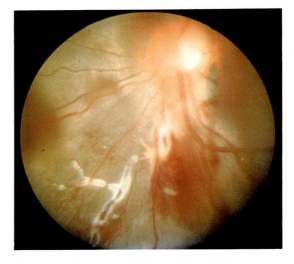

Figure 1.20 Severe periphlebitis with 'candlewax drippings' and vitreous haemorrhage (courtesy of Mr J. Shilling)

Differential diagnosis

It is important to remember that tumours may occasionally present with inflammatory signs which may be mistaken for endogenous uveitis (masquerade syndromes).

Retinoblastoma

In all young children with uveitis it is extremely important to exclude the possibility of a retinoblastoma, which may mimic a posterior uveitis or cause a 'pseudo-hypopyon'; very rarely it may invade the iris and give rise to 'pseudo-Busacca nodules' (*Figure 1.21*).

Melanoma

A necrotizing malignant melanoma may also give rise to a 'pseudo-uveitis'.

Histiocytic lymphoma (reticulum cell sarcoma)

This very rare tumour should be considered in the differential diagnosis of chronic vitritis in patients between the ages of 40 and 60 years. The fundus shows yellow subretinal and choroidal infiltrates, frequently with multiple hyperpigmented spots.

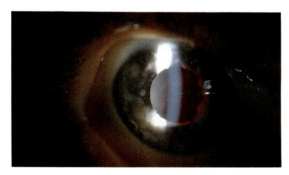

Figure 1.21 Retinoblastoma invading iris giving rise to 'pseudo-Busacca' nodules

Further reading

HOGAN, M.J., KIMURA, S.J. and THYGESON, P. (1959) Signs and symptoms of uveitis. 1. Anterior uveitis. *American Journal of Ophthalmology*, **47**, 155–170

KIMURA, S.J., THYGESON, P. and HOGAN, M.J. (1959) Signs and symptoms of uveitis. 2. Classification of posterior manifestations of uveitis. *American Journal of Ophthalmology*, **47**, 171–176

NUSSENBLATT, R.B., PALESTINE, A.G., CHAN, C-C. *et al.* (1985) Standardization of vitreal inflammatory activity in intermediate and posterior uveitis. *Ophthalmology*, **92**, 467–471

2

Arthritis

Ankylosing spondylitis

Systemic features

Ankylosing spondylitis (AS) is a chronic inflammatory arthritis of unknown aetiology that predominantly affects the axial skeleton. The disease typically affects males between the ages of 20 and 40 years who are positive for HLA-B27 but negative for rheumatoid factor ('seronegative'). The initial symptom of AS is morning stiffness or aching of the lower back which improves with activity. In advanced cases bony ankylosis may cause a fixed flexion deformity of the spine and some patients also develop cardiovascular complications, notably aortic incompetence. In females, AS has a more benign course than in males and in children the disease frequently presents with a peripheral lower limb arthropathy without backache. Some patients with AS also have ulcerative colitis or Crohn's disease.

Diagnostic tests

X-rays

All young adult males with acute unilateral iridocyclitis should have X-rays of the sacro-iliac joints irrespective of the presence or absence of low back symptoms. This is because in early cases the X-rays may be positive before the patient is symptomatic. The diagnosis of subclinical AS is important because appropriate therapy may prevent the development of more severe structural changes in the spine.

> *Note* More sensitive methods such as radioactive scanning using technetium may demonstrate active sacro-iliitis in patients with normal X-rays.

Tissue typing

Between 80 and 90% of patients with AS are positive for HLA-B27, as opposed to an incidence of about 8% in the general population. The incidence of HLA-B27 in patients with acute iridocyclitis is about 45% and in those with both AS and acute iridocyclitis, the incidence rises to about 95%. The presence of HLA-B27 in a patient with early X-ray findings, therefore, merely confirms the diagnosis of AS. Patients with acute anterior uveitis, who are positive for HLA-B27 but radiologically normal, should be examined by a rheumatologist at two-yearly intervals for evidence of sacro-iliac involvement as there is a strong likelihood that they will eventually develop AS.

> *Note* Tests for rheumatoid factor (Rose Waaler, DAT) are of no diagnostic value as they are always negative in AS.

Ocular features

The typical ocular complication of AS is an acute, recurrent, non-granulomatous iridocyclitis. The active inflammation is invariably unilateral although both eyes are frequently involved at different times. The incidence of acute iridocyclitis in patients with AS is 30% and conversely about 30% of males with acute unilateral iridocyclitis will also have AS. However, there is no correlation between the severity and activity of eye and joint involvement and uveitis may either precede or follow the diagnosis of AS.

Symptoms

The symptoms are those of an acute unilateral anterior uveitis.

Signs

External   Diffuse ciliary injection is present and the pupil is small (*Figure 1.2*).

Slitlamp   Initially the corneal endothelium shows 'dusting' (*Figure 1.4*) and later small keratic precipitates may form. The aqueous contains many cells (usually between +3 and +4) as well as a flare (*Figure 2.1*). In severe cases the anterior chamber contains a fibrinous exudate (*Figure 2.2*) which also coats the anterior lens surface and a hypopyon (*Figure 2.3*) may also be seen.

Vitreous   The anterior vitreous contains many cells.

Fundus   This is usually normal although mild macular oedema develops in a few cases.

Clinical course and complications

The attack of iridocyclitis seldom lasts longer than 6 weeks. The main complication is the formation of posterior synechiae (*Figure 2.4*) which, if severe,

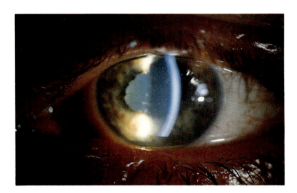

Figure 2.1 Aqueous cells (+4), dense flare and posterior synechiae in recurrent anterior uveitis associated with ankylosing spondylitis

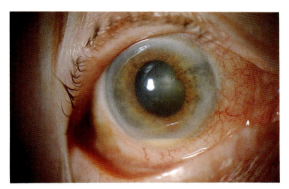

Figure 2.3 Hypopyon

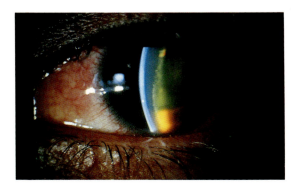

Figure 2.2 Fibrinous exudate in anterior chamber

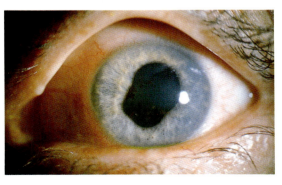

Figure 2.4 Extensive posterior synechiae and pigment on anterior lens surface following an attack of acute anterior uveitis

may lead to secondary glaucoma from iris bombè. Although there is a high risk that the uveitis will recur in one or other eye, the long-term visual prognosis is good and vision-threatening complications such as secondary cataract and chronic cystoid macular oedema are rare. In a few patients with many recurrent attacks the inflammation eventually becomes chronic.

Management

The treatment of acute iridocyclitis is with topical or periocular steroids and mydriatics. Details of treatment are discussed in Chapter 10.

Differential diagnosis

Other causes of acute iridocyclitis include Reiter's syndrome, psoriatic arthritis, Behçet's disease, sarcoidosis and the syndrome of acute anterior uveitis in young adults.

Reiter's syndrome

Systemic features

Reiter's syndrome consists of a triad of urethritis, conjunctivitis and 'seronegative' arthritis. This relatively uncommon disease which typically affects young men, 70% of whom are positive for HLA-B27, has three modes of presentation.

1 *Postvenereal* The most common presentation is with a non-specific (i.e. non-gonococcal) urethritis, 2 weeks following sexual intercourse. Chlamydial infection has been implicated as a cause of this form of Reiter's syndrome.
2 *Postdysenteric* A less common presentation is following an attack of dysentery without a preliminary urethritis.
3 *Articular* In some patients, acute arthritis is the first feature of the disease, with either urethritis or dysentery being insignificant. The inflammation typically affects the knees, ankles, and Achilles tendon. A periostitis may cause a calcaneal spur and some patients subsequently develop ankylosing spondylitis.

Other systemic features of Reiter's syndrome include keratoderma blennorrhagica of the palms or soles, circinate balanitis, nail dystrophy, mouth ulceration and plantar fasciitis.

> *Note* The mouth ulcers are usually painless in contrast to the painful aphthous stomatitis of Behçet's disease.

Reiter's syndrome is a chronic disease characterized by remissions and recurrences. The initial attack may last several weeks or months and various parts of the syndrome may recur during the ensuing years.

Diagnostic tests

X-rays The knees, ankles, heels, feet and sacro-iliac joints may show asymptomatic arthritis.

Tissue typing Patients with uveitis are usually positive for HLA-B27.

Cultures *Chlamydia trachomatis* may be isolated from the conjunctiva and urethra of affected individuals. Isolation of *Salmonella*, *Shigella*, and *Yersinia* from faeces may also be helpful in establishing the diagnosis.

Blood tests The white cell count and erythrocyte sedimentation rate (ESR) are usually raised during active disease.

Ocular features

Conjunctivitis Although a mucopurulent conjunctivitis without follicles is common it is not universal. It usually follows the urethritis by about 2 weeks, and it typically precedes the arthritis.

Keratitis A punctate epithelial or subepithelial keratitis with anterior stromal infiltrates (*Figure 2.5*) may accompany the conjunctival inflammation.

Iridocyclitis An acute unilateral iridocyclitis occurs in about 20% of patients, either with the first attack of Reiter's syndrome or during a recurrence.

Psoriatic arthritis

Systemic features

Psoriatic arthritis is a 'seronegative', anodular, erosive, inflammatory arthritis occurring in about 5% of patients with psoriasis. The disease has no sexual preferential but is associated with an increased prevalence of HLA-B27 and HLA-B17. Typically, the arthritis is asymmetrical and involves the interphalangeal joints of the hands and feet. In some cases the sacro-iliac joints and the spine are also affected. Many patients show the typical nail pitting of psoriasis.

Ocular features

Conjunctivitis   About 20% of patients develop conjunctivitis.

Keratoconjunctivitis sicca   This is a relatively rare complication.

> *Note*   Psoriatic arthritis is the only seronegative spondyloarthritis that may be associated with dry eyes.

Keratitis   Some patients with anterior uveitis develop raised corneal infiltrates just inside the limbus.

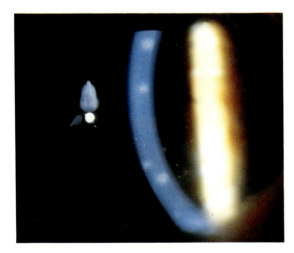

Figure 2.5 Keratitis in Reiter's syndrome

Iridocyclitis   An acute unilateral iridocyclitis occurs less frequently in psoriatic arthritis than in either ankylosing spondylitis or Reiter's syndrome.

Differential diagnosis

There are several similarities between Reiter's syndrome and psoriatic arthritis. They are both associated with skin and nail changes as well as sacro-iliitis and acute iridocyclitis.

Juvenile chronic arthritis

Systemic features

Juvenile chronic arthritis (JCA) is a 'seronegative' idiopathic inflammatory arthritis developing in children under the age of 16 years. In the United States, the disease is frequently referred to as 'juvenile rheumatoid arthritis'. Based on the mode of onset of the disease and the extent of joint involvement during the first three months, three different subgroups of JCA are recognized.

Systemic onset JCA

Systemic onset JCA, which accounts for about 30% of cases, is characterized by a high remittent fever and at least one of the following features: transient maculopapular rash, generalized lymphadenopathy, hepatomegaly, splenomegaly, and pericarditis. Initially, arthralgia or arthritis may be absent or minimal and only a minority of patients subsequently develop a progressive polyarthritis.

> *Note*   The term 'Still's disease' is now usually reserved for patients in this subgroup, in which uveitis is extremely rare.

Polyarticular onset JCA

Polyarticular onset JCA accounts for about 20% of all cases. The disease affects five or more joints during the first three months. The most frequently involved joints are the knees followed by the wrists and ankles. In some patients, the arthritis persists for many years and causes crippling deformities.

Note   Uveitis is fairly rare in this subgroup.

Pauciarticular onset JCA

Pauciarticular onset JCA is the most frequent accounting for about 50% of all cases. In this subgroup, four or fewer joints are involved during the first three months. The most commonly affected joints are the knees (*Figure 2.6*), although occasionally the arthritis involves only a single finger or toe. Some patients in this subgroup remain pauciarticular whilst others subsequently develop a polyarthritis.

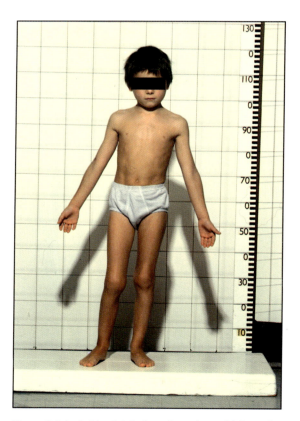

Figure 2.6 Arthritis of right knee in patient with juvenile chronic arthritis (courtesy of Dr B. Ansell)

Note
1 About 25% of patients in this subgroup develop uveitis.
2 Seventy-five per cent of all patients with JCA and uveitis are girls.

Diagnostic tests

Rheumatoid factor   All patients with uveitis and JCA are seronegative for rheumatoid factor. This confirms the fact that seropositive children with 'true' juvenile rheumatoid arthritis resemble their adult counterparts and are not at increased risk of uveitis.

Note   Routine screening of the eyes of children with 'true' seropositive juvenile rheumatoid arthritis is therefore unnecessary.

Antinuclear antibodies (ANA)   About 75% of children with JCA and uveitis are positive for ANA as compared to an incidence of 30% in those without ocular involvement. It has been suggested that ANA formation precedes rather than follows the onset of uveitis and that a rising titre should arouse suspicion as to the increased risk of uveitis. However, there is no correlation between the level of ANA titre and the severity of either eye or joint disease.

Note   Thirty per cent of patients with the syndrome of juvenile chronic iridocyclitis, who do not have arthritis, are also ANA positive (*see* Chapter 8).

In about 50% of children, the interval between the onset of JCA and uveitis is 2 years or less and only 10% of patients develop uveitis after 7 years. There is no correlation between the activity of joint and eye involvement.

Note   Six per cent of children develop uveitis before arthritis.

Because the onset of intraocular inflammation is invariably *asymptomatic*, it is extremely important for children at risk to have regular *slitlamp biomicroscopy*. The frequency of examination is governed by the various risk factors just discussed which are summarized in *Table 2.1*.

Table 2.1 Risk factors for JCA

Onset of JCA	Risk of uveitis	Examination frequency
Systemic	±	Annual
Polyarticular	+	9-monthly
Polyarticular + ANA	++	6-monthly
Pauciarticular	+++	4-monthly
Pauciarticular + ANA	++++	3-monthly

Clinical features

The anterior uveitis in JCA is chronic, non-granulomatous and bilateral in 70% of cases. It is unusual for patients with initially unilateral uveitis to develop involvement of the second eye after more than one year. In those with bilateral uveitis, the severity of intraocular inflammation is usually symmetrical.

Symptoms

As the onset of intraocular inflammation is invariably asymptomatic, the uveitis is frequently detected on routine slitlamp examination. Even during acute exacerbations with +4 cells in the aqueous humour, it is rare for patients to complain, although a few report an increase in vitreous floaters.

Signs

External The eye is white, even in the presence of severe uveitis.

Slitlamp The keratic precipitates are usually small to medium in size. During acute exacerbations the entire corneal endothelium shows 'dusting' by many hundreds of cells (*Figure 1.4*) but hypopyon is very rare.

Note 'Endothelial dusting' is a particularly useful sign of exacerbation when adequate slitlamp examination of the aqueous cannot be performed in a young and uncooperative child.

Posterior synechiae are common in eyes with long-standing undetected uveitis. In some eyes the iris surface shows dilated blood vessels which may extend onto the lens. Although the intraocular inflammation is essentially non-granulomatous, some eyes show small Koeppe nodules. Pigment deposition on the anterior lens surface is common and some eyes also have pupillary tags (*Figure 2.7*).

Vitreous Cells in the anterior vitreous are common.

Fundus A few eyes develop chronic cystoid macular oedema.

Clinical course and complications (Figure 2.8)

The severity of uveitis can be divided into four groups:

1 In about 10% of cases the intraocular inflammation is very mild, unassociated with keratic precipitates, with never more than +1 aqueous cells and persists for less than 12 months.
2 About 15% of patients have one attack of uveitis which lasts less than 4 months, with the severity

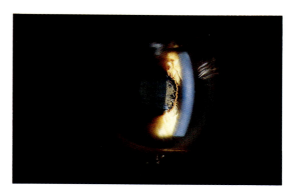

Figure 2.7 Pupillary tags and pigment on anterior lens surface

(a)

(b)

(c)

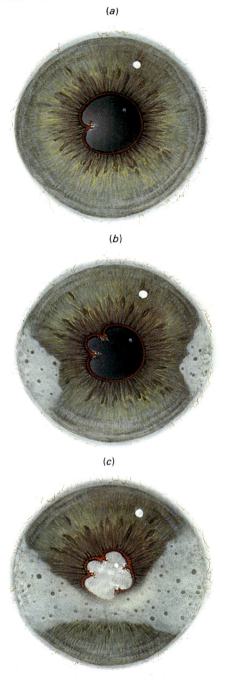

Figure 2.8 Progression of complications of chronic iridocyclitis associated with juvenile chronic arthritis: (a) posterior synechiae, (b) increase in number of posterior synechiae and early band keratopathy, (c) extensive band keratopathy and mature complicated cataract

of inflammation varying from +2 to +4 aqueous cells.

3 In 50% of cases, the uveitis is moderate to severe and persists for more than 4 months. The majority of acute exacerbations can be controlled by frequent instillation of topical steroids.

4 In 25% of cases, the intraocular inflammation is very severe, lasts for several years and responds poorly to treatment. In this subgroup, band keratopathy occurs in 40% of patients, complicated cataract in 30%, and secondary inflammatory glaucoma in 15%.

Management of uveitis

Most patients can be controlled with topical steroids. Those that respond poorly to topical medication are also frequently resistant to systemic steroid therapy although they may respond to periocular injections. The therapeutic value of cytotoxic agents such as chlorambucil is undetermined. Details of management of chronic anterior uveitis are discussed in Chapter 10.

Management of band keratopathy

The band keratopathy initially appears as subepithelial opacities just inside the limbus at 3 and 9 o'clock. The opacities may remain localized but frequently they extend centrally to coalesce just below the centre of the pupil and then spread irregularly upwards in the interpalpebral area of the cornea. The band keratopathy frequently becomes chalky in appearance and, with a slitlamp, holes can be seen within the opacity which are thought to represent nerve canals in Bowman's layer of the cornea.

Removal of band keratopathy is indicated when the visual axis is obstructed, or when adequate visualization of the anterior segment is impossible. The calcium salts are readily abstracted from the cornea by chelation as follows:

1 The corneal epithelium overlying the opacity is scraped off with a knife (*Figure 2.9*).

2 A 0.01 M solution of sodium versenate (disodium ethylenediaminetetraacetic acid) is applied to the cornea with a cotton-tipped bud (*Figure 2.10*), until all calcium has been removed. This usually takes about 10 minutes. Recurrences of band keratopathy are rare even if the uveitis persists.

Differential diagnosis

Masquerade syndrome It is extremely important to exclude the possibility of retinoblastoma in all children with 'uveitis'.

Juvenile spondylitis (JS) In children, the distinction between early JS and JCA may be difficult. This is because children with JS seldom complain of backache or sciatic pain and X-rays of the sacro-iliac joints are frequently normal because the disease invariably presents with a peripheral lower limb arthritis. Patients with JS are usually boys who develop arthritis at around the age of 10 years and, just like their adult counterparts, they have a very high prevalence of HLA-B27. The typical presenting ocular feature in JS is a unilateral symptomatic acute anterior uveitis, although a few subsequently develop a bilateral chronic iridocyclitis identical to that seen in JCA.

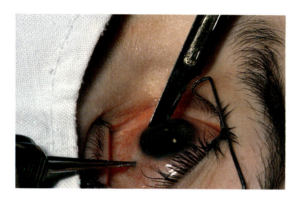

Figure 2.9 Removal of corneal epithelium with knife

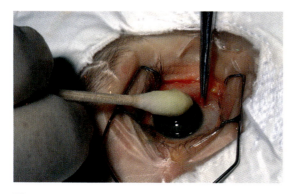

Figure 2.10 Application of sodium versenate to cornea

Sarcoidosis Although sarcoidosis is very rare in children it may occasionally present with an anterior uveitis and arthropathy.

Idiopathic juvenile chronic iridocyclitis The vast majority of children with chronic iridocyclitis do not have an associated systemic disease although the clinical features of the intraocular inflammation and complications are the same as in JCA.

Further reading

Ankylosing spondylitis
BECKINSALE, A.B., DAVIES, J., GIBSON, J.M. *et al.* (1984) Acute anterior uveitis, ankylosing spondylitis, back pain, and HLA-B27. *British Journal of Ophthalmology,* **68,** 741–745

BECKINSALE, A.B., GUSS, R.B. and ROSENTHAL, A.R. (1982) Acute anterior uveitis associated with HLA-B27 positive tissue type. A comparative study of two populations. *Transactions of the Ophthalmological Society of the United Kingdom,* **102,** 168–170

BREWERTON, D.A. (1985) The genetics of acute anterior uveitis. *Transactions of the Ophthalmological Society of the United Kingdom,* **104,** 248–249

BREWERTON, D.A., CAFFREY, M., HART, F.D. *et al.* (1973a) Ankylosing spondylitis and HLA-B27. *Lancet,* **i,** 904–907

BREWERTON, D.A., CAFFREY, M., NICHOLLS, A. *et al.* (1973b) Acute anterior uveitis and HLA-B27. *Lancet,* **ii,** 994–996

KIMURA, S.J., HOGAN, M.J., O'CONNOR, G.R. *et al.* (1967) Uveitis and joint disease. *Archives of Ophthalmology,* **77,** 309–316

OHNO, S., KIMURA, S.J., O'CONNOR, G.R. *et al.* (1977) HLA antigens and uveitis. *British Journal of Ophthalmology,* **61,** 62–64

Reiter's disease
PURCELL, J.J.JR, BALDASSARE, A.R. and TSAI, C.C. (1980) Reiter's syndrome. *Perspectives in Ophthalmology,* **4,** 17–22

Juvenile chronic arthritis
KANSKI, J.J. (1977) Anterior uveitis in juvenile rheumatoid arthritis. *Archives of Ophthalmology,* **95,** 1794–1797

KANSKI, J.J. (1981) Care of children with anterior uveitis. *Transactions of the Ophthalmological Society of the United Kingdom,* **101,** 387–390

KANSKI, J.J. and SHUN-SHIN, G.A. (1984) Systemic uveitis syndromes in childhood: An analysis of 360 cases. *Ophthalmology,* **91,** 1247–1251

KEY, S.N. and KIMURA, S.J. (1975) Iridocyclitis associated with juvenile rheumatoid arthritis. *American Journal of Ophthalmology,* **80,** 425–429

PALMER, R.G., KANSKI, J.J. and ANSELL, B.M. (1985)

Chlorambucil in the treatment of intractable uveitis associated with juvenile chronic arthritis. *Journal of Rheumatology*, **12**, 967–970

PERKINS, E.S. (1966) Patterns of uveitis in children. *British Journal of Ophthalmology*, **50**, 169–185

SCHALLER, J.G., JOHNSON, G.D., HOLBOROW, E.J. *et al.* (1974) The association of antinuclear antibodies with the chronic iridocyclitis in juvenile rheumatoid arthritis (Still's disease). *Arthritis and Rheumatism*, **17**, 409–416

SMILEY, W.K. (1974). The eye in juvenile rheumatoid arthritis. *Transactions of the Ophthalmological Society of the United Kingdom*, **94**, 817–829

3

Non-infectious systemic diseases

Sarcoidosis

Systemic features

The definition of sarcoidosis proposed by the Seventh International Conference on Sarcoidosis and other Granulomatous Disorders is as follows:

Sarcoidosis is a multisystem granulomatous disorder of unknown aetiology, most commonly affecting young adults and presenting most frequently with bilateral hilar lymphadenopathy, pulmonary infiltration, skin, and eye lesions. The diagnosis is established most securely when clinicoradiographic findings are supported by histological evidence of widespread non-caseating epithelioid-cell granulomas in more than one organ or a positive Kveim–Slitzbach skin test. Immunological features are depression of delayed-type hypersensitivity suggesting impaired cell-mediated immunity and raised or abnormal immunoglobulins. There may also be hypercalciuria, with or without hypercalcaemia. The course and prognosis may correlate with the mode of onset: an acute onset with erythema nodosum (*Figure 3.1*) heralds a self-limiting course and spontaneous resolution, whereas an insidious onset may be followed by relentless, progressive fibrosis. Corticosteroids relieve symptoms and suppress inflammation and granuloma formation.

> *Note* Sarcoidosis usually presents during the third and fourth decades and is more common in Blacks and females.

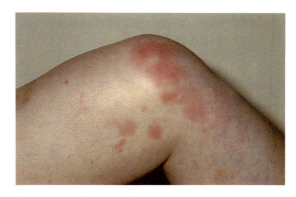

Figure 3.1 Erythema nodosum

Diagnostic tests

Although the diagnosis is usually easy, in some patients many of the features are missing and the following special investigations may be useful.

Chest X-ray (Figure 3.2) Over 90% of patients with ocular sarcoid will have an abnormal chest X-ray. The most common initial finding is bilateral hilar fullness (stage 1). This is followed by the appearance of reticulonodular infiltrates (stage 2). The hilar involvement then wanes and only pulmonary fibrosis remains (stage 3).

Biopsy Lung biopsy by the tracheobronchial fibreoptic technique is now frequently carried out and is accurate in about 90% of patients in diagnosing sarcoidosis. Biopsy of lacrimal gland, conjunctiva, lymph nodes, tonsil and liver may also give histological confirmation of sarcoidosis.

Note Transconjunctival biopsy of the palpebral portion of the lacrimal gland is safe and should be considered in patients with suspected sarcoidosis, particularly if the lacrimal glands are enlarged or demonstrate increased gallium localization. Biopsies are positive in 25% of patients with unenlarged lacrimal glands and in 75% of cases with lacrimal gland enlargement.

Broncheoalveolar lavage This lavage with analysis of the fluid for T-lymphocytes is a relatively new test.

Kveim–Slitzbach test This is positive in 80% of patients with sarcoidosis. It relies on the fact that a saline suspension of sarcoid tissue (antigen) obtained from the spleen of a patient with active sarcoidosis, introduced intradermally induces a granuloma of sarcoid type when biopsied 4 weeks later. However, the reaction is suppressed by systemic steroids. The main disadvantage of this test is the difficulty in obtaining the antigen as it is not commercially available. In addition care must be taken to exclude a non-specific foreign body reaction when the skin lesion is examined histologically.

Mantoux test Although this is negative in a very high percentage of patients with sarcoidosis, it is now of limited value except in areas with a high incidence of positive tuberculin tests.

Angiotensin converting enzyme (ACE) ACE is produced by many cells in the body. In sarcoidosis the enzyme is thought to be synthesized by monocytes that have transformed from phagocytic into storage or secretory cells. Normal serum levels of ACE are 12–35 nmol/min per μl in men and 11–29 nmol/min per μl in women. Serum ACE is usually elevated in patients with active sarcoidosis and is normal in patients in remission. Because patients with active ocular sarcoidosis may be in systemic remission, the test has serious sensitivity deficiencies. The test also has serious specificity deficiencies because the serum ACE level may also be raised in other conditions such as tuberculosis, carcinomatosis, histoplasmosis, rheumatoid arthritis, ankylosing spondylitis etc., some of which are also associated with intraocular inflammation.

Calcium Calcium metabolism is abnormal in sarcoidosis and hypercalciuria is common (although hypercalcaemia is unusual).

Serum lysozyme This is elevated in patients with active systemic sarcoidosis. Unfortunately, just like ACE, it is also raised in other systemic diseases.

Gallium-67 scan of head, neck and thorax This frequently shows increased uptake in patients with active systemic sarcoidosis because the gallium is taken up by mitotically active liposomes of granulocytes.

Ocular features

The eye is involved in about 30% of patients with systemic sarcoidosis. Ocular involvement may

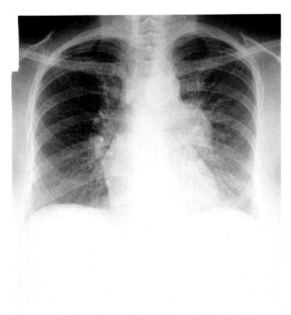

Figure 3.2 Hilar adenopathy and lung infiltration in sarcoidosis (courtesy of Mr M. Sanders)

occur in patients with few, if any, constitutional symptoms, as well as in those with inactive systemic disease. Indeed, like tuberculosis and syphilis, the diagnosis may be missed for long periods of time and, in fact, sarcoidosis has now replaced syphilis as the 'great imitator'. In acute sarcoidosis the ocular inflammation is usually unilateral and, as the disease becomes chronic, bilateral involvement usually develops.

Signs

External (Figure 3.3) Sarcoidosis may involve the conjunctiva, the episclera, and rarely the orbit and sclera. The skin of the eyelids may show violaceous sarcoid plaques (lupus pernio). Sarcoid granulomas of the lid margins may be mistaken for small chalazia. Granulomatous infiltration of the lacrimal gland, if severe, may be responsible for keratoconjunctivitis sicca.

Slitlamp Iridocyclitis is by far the most common ocular complication, it may be acute or chronic.

Acute iridocyclitis, which is frequently unilateral, typically affects young patients with acute sarcoidosis.

Chronic granulomatous iridocyclitis, which is frequently bilateral, is more common than the acute form. It typically affects older patients with chronic lung fibrosis in whom the systemic disease may be inactive. The intraocular inflammation may be difficult to control and complications such as band keratopathy, complicated cataract and secondary glaucoma are frequent.

Note About 5% of all cases of anterior uveitis are caused by sarcoidosis

Vitreous

Diffuse vitritis is common, and more dense inferiorly.

Nodules—see retinal involvement.

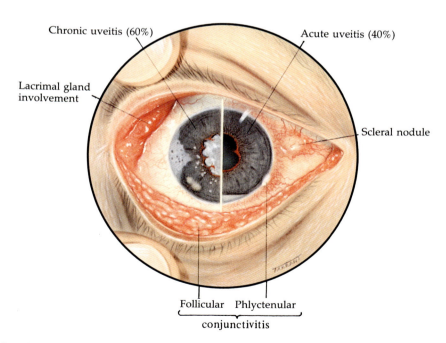

Figure 3.3 Anterior segment complications of sarcoidosis

Haemorrhage may be secondary to new vessels on the optic disc or in the retinal periphery.

Fundus (Figure 3.4) The posterior segment is involved in about 25% of patients with ocular sarcoid and is usually associated with anterior uveitis. The posterior segment manifestations are caused by granulomatous penetration of the retinal and choroidal vessels with secondary damage involving: (1) the blood vessels, (2) the retina, (3) the choroid, and (4) the optic nerve.

Blood vessels The most subtle and common sign of posterior segment sarcoidosis is a peripheral retinal periphlebitis involving only one or two segments of a retinal vein. Active periphlebitis is characterized by soft, white, perivenous infiltration (cuffing) associated with increased vascular permeability which may lead to peripheral globular retinal haemorrhages and intraretinal oedema. The acute lesions stain on fundus fluorescein angiography. Although acute periphlebitis may resolve spontaneously or with the use of systemic steroids, vascular sheathing, once established,

usually persists. An advanced stage of periphlebitis caused by perivascular accumulation of granulomatous tissue (periphlebitic nodules) is known as 'candlewax drippings' (*see Figure 1.20*). Two complications of periphlebitis are retinal branch vein occlusion (*Figure 3.5*) and peripheral 'seafan' neovascularization (fronds).

> *Note* Inactive perivasculitis is recognized as grey-white vascular sheathing without retinal haemorrhage or oedema which does not stain on fundus fluorescein angiography.

Retina The 'spillover' of granulomatous tissue may result in retinal granulomas which may be associated with secondary neovascularization. In advanced cases, the sarcoid nodules may be located on the retinal surface and they may also extend into the vitreous. Preretinal nodules are typically discrete, grey-white, and located inferiorly and anterior to the equator (Landers' sign)

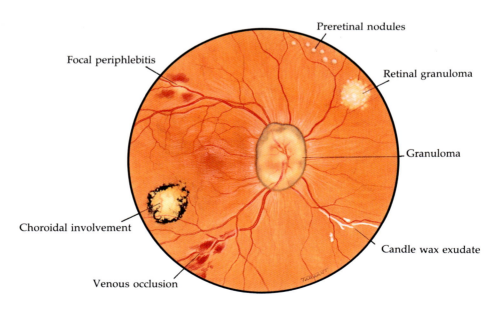

Figure 3.4 Posterior segment complications of sarcoidosis

(*Figure 3.6*). The most severe form of retinal sarcoid is called 'acute sarcoid retinopathy' which is characterized by a vitreous haze, candlewax drippings, retinal and preretinal granulomas, and retinal haemorrhages.

Choroid Choroidal sarcoidosis is relatively rare and is usually not associated with retinal or vitreous inflammation. The choroidal granulomas are typically bilateral, multiple, pale-yellow, elevated lesions at the posterior pole. They vary in size from small subpigment epithelial granulomas to large choroidal masses. Visual acuity may be reduced due to secondary elevation of the sensory retina at the fovea. Occasionally the lesions may be associated with the formation of subretinal neovascular membranes.

Optic nerve Sarcoidosis may give rise to the following lesions of the optic nerve:

1 Focal granulomas may involve the optic nerve head but do not usually affect visual acuity.
2 Papilloedema is usually secondary to extensive involvement of the central nervous system and it may occur in the absence of other ocular lesions.

3 Neovascularization of the optic nerve head is an occasional complication of retinal branch vein occlusion secondary to severe periphlebitis or, rarely, it may be associated with an optic nerve head granuloma.

Management

Most ocular complications can be treated by topical and/or periocular steroids. Systemic steroids may be necessary in patients with severe posterior segment disease, particularly if the optic nerve is involved. Fundus neovascualrization can be treated by laser photocoagulation provided the intraocular inflammation is adequately controlled.

Differential diagnosis

Tuberculosis Both anterior and posterior segment findings may be similar.

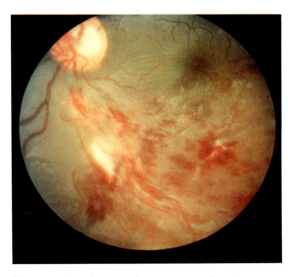

Figure 3.5 Branch vein occlusion in sarcoidosis (courtesy of Mr J. Shilling)

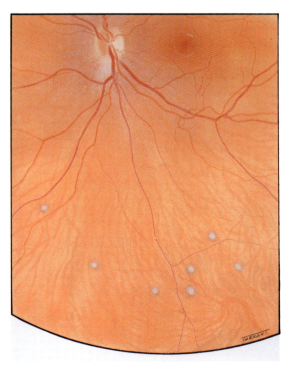

Figure 3.6 Preretinal nodules in sarcoidosis (Landers' sign)

Sickle-cell retinopathy In Black patients the peripheral 'seafan' neovascularization may be mistaken for proliferative sickle-cell retinopathy.

Pars planitis The preretinal nodules of sarcoid may be mistaken for the 'snowballs' of pars planitis. Both conditions are associated with a periphlebitis and vitritis.

Choroidal metastasis A large choroidal sarcoid granuloma may resemble a choroidal metastasis.

Eales' disease (idiopathic retinal vasculitis) The retinal periphlebitis of sarcoidosis is similar to that seen in Eales' disease (*see* Chapter 9).

Behçet's disease

Systemic features

Behçet's disease is an idiopathic multisystem disease which typically affects young men from the eastern Mediterranean region and Japan who are positive for HLA-B5. The basic lesion is an obliterative vasculitis probably caused by abnormal circulating immune complexes. The four 'major' features of Behçet's disease are the following:

1 Recurrent oral ulceration is a universal finding and, in the majority of patients, the presenting sign. The aphthous ulcers are painful and shallow with a central yellowish necrotic base. They tend to occur in crops and may involve the tongue, gums, lips (*Figure 3.7*) and buccal mucosa.

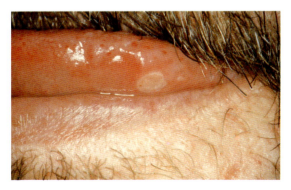

Figure 3.7 Lip ulcer in Behçet's disease

> *Note* The oral ulceration in Reiter's syndrome is painless.

2 Genital ulceration is present in about 90% of patients and is more obvious and troublesome in men than in women.
3 Skin lesions which include erythema nodosum (*Figure 3.1*), pustules, cutaneous hypersensitivity, and ulceration.
4 Uveitis.

The six 'minor' features of Behçet's disease are the following:

1 Thrombophlebitis which may involve the superficial veins or the vena cavae.
2 Arthritis which is asymmetrical, nondestructive, and typically affects the knees.
3 Gastrointestinal lesions in the form of peptic ulceration and colitis.
4 Central nervous system involvement (which may be fatal) in the form of mental changes, mid-brain lesions, transverse myelitis of the spinal cord, cranial nerve palsies and meningoencephalitis.
5 Cardiovascular lesions such as pericarditis, arterial occlusions and aneurysms.
6 A positive family history.

Since there are no specific confirmatory diagnostic laboratory tests the diagnosis of Behçet's disease requires the presence of at least three 'major' lesions, or two 'major' and at least two 'minor'.

> *Note* About 50% of patients with Behçet's disease develop a 'tuberculin-like' reaction after an intradermal puncture with a hypodermic needle or an injection of 0.1 ml of saline intradermally. Some patients may develop a small skin pustule following this procedure.

Ocular features

About 70% of patients with Behçet's disease develop recurrent bilateral, non-granulomatous intraocular inflammation. In any individual patients, either anterior or posterior segment involvement can predominate.

Signs

External   Conjunctivitis, episcleritis, and keratitis (*Figure 3.8*) occur in a few patients.

Slitlamp   Acute recurrent iridocyclitis which may be associated with a transient hypopyon is common.

Vitreous   Vitritis which may be severe and persistent is universal in eyes with uveitis.

Fundus   The posterior segment changes can be of three main types (*Figure 3.9*):

1 Diffuse vascular leakage throughout the fundus is the most common and persistent finding. It

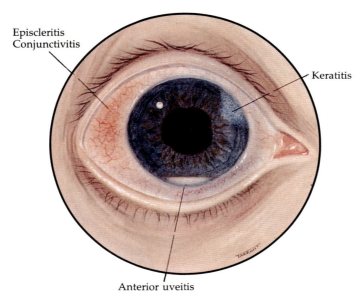

Figure 3.8 Anterior segment complications of Behçet's disease

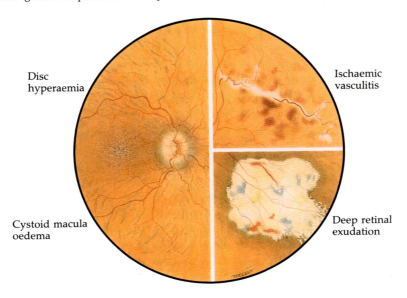

Figure 3.9 Posterior segment complications of Behçet's disease

frequently gives rise to diffuse retinal oedema, cystoid macular oedema, and occasionally oedema or hyperaemia of the optic disc.

2 Retinal vasculitis predominantly involving the veins (periphlebitis) is also frequent. In severe cases it caused occlusion of major retinal veins which may subsequently lead to neovascularization.

3 Retinitis, in the form of white necrotic infiltrates of the inner retina which may be associated with intraretinal haemorrhages, may be seen during the active stages of the systemic disease. The infiltrates are usually transient and do not lead to secondary scarring. In some patients, however, acute massive retinal exudation involving the outer retinal layers with associated obliteration of the overlying blood vessels leads to areas of retinal necrosis and atrophy.

Clinical course and complications

The uveitis associated with Behçet's disease has a relatively poor visual prognosis. The acute iridocyclitis may become chronic and lead to phthisis bulbi (*Figure 3.10*). Posterior segment involvement may lead to severe attenuation of the retinal vasculature (*Figure 3.11*) and blindness from secondary optic atrophy.

Management

Initially the acute anterior uveitis usually responds well to topical steroid therapy. However, posterior segment involvement is frequently unresponsive to systemic steroid medication although in some cases are sensitive to chlorambucil (*see* Chapter 10).

Vogt–Koyanagi–Harada syndrome

Systemic features

The Vogt–Koyanagi–Harada (V-K-H) syndrome is an idiopathic, multisystem disorder which typically affects pigmented individuals. Japanese patients, in whom the disorder is relatively common, have an increased prevalence of HLA-B22. In order to establish the diagnosis of V-K-H, at least three of the following four groups of signs must be present:

1 Cutaneous signs

Alopecia (baldness) occurs in about 60% of patients and is usually confined to small areas.

Poliosis (whitening of eyelashes) is also common and usually develops several weeks after the onset of the disease.

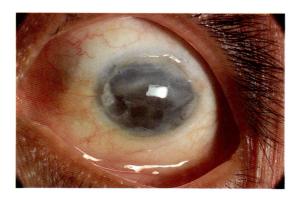

Figure 3.10 Phthisis bulbi

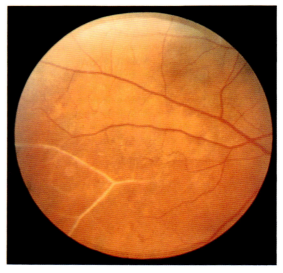

Figure 3.11 Vascular occlusion in Behçet's disease (courtesy Mr A. Shun-Shin)

Vitiligo (patches of skin depigmentation) (*Figure 3.12*) usually follows the onset of visual symptoms by several weeks.

2 Neurological signs

Neurological irritation, such as headache and stiffness develop simultaneously with ocular involvement.

Encephalopathy is less frequent than meningeal involvement. It may be manifest as convulsions, cranial nerve palsies, and paresis.

Auditory symptoms include tinnitus, vertigo, and deafness.

Cerebrospinal fluid lymphocytosis is present during the acute phase of the disorder.

3 Anterior uveitis This is bilateral and chronic.

4 Posterior uveitis This includes exudative retinal detachment.

> *Note* The full V-K-H syndrome probably reflects the integration of the Vogt–Koyanagi syndrome with Harada's disease. In the former, anterior uveitis predominates and skin and hair changes are common, wheras Harada's disease is characterized mainly by meningeal irritation and posterior segment involvement.

Ocular features

Symptoms

These depend on the site of initial involvement. Although both eyes are usually affected, one may become involved several days or weeks before the other.

Signs

External In eyes with anterior uveitis the eye may show ciliary injection.

Slitlamp A granulomatous iridocyclitis is present.

Vitreous A vitritis is present in all eyes.

Fundus Posterior segment involvement usually starts with the appearance of a multifocal choroiditis (*Figure 3.13*) which may be associated with disc hyperaemia or oedema. Later, exudative retinal detachments develop which may be either extensive and bullous or relatively flat and confined to the posterior pole.

Clinical course and complications

Anterior uveitis This has a chronic course and frequently leads to posterior synechiae, secondary glaucoma and cataract.

Posterior uveitis The exudative retinal detachments gradually subside either spontaneously or with the help of systemic steroids leaving mottled scars corresponding to atrophy and proliferation

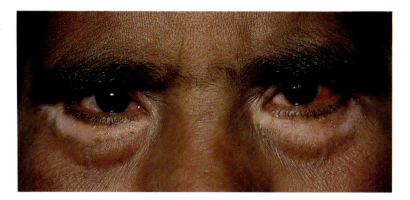

Figure 3.12 Vitiligo

of the retinal pigment epithelium. Visual acuity may remain good even with involvement of the macula.

> *Note*   In contrast to the anterior uveitis, posterior segment recurrences do not occur.

Management

Anterior uveitis is treated vigorously with topical steroids and, if necessary, also with periocular and systemic therapy. The exudative retinal detachments may settle after only a few days of systemic steroid therapy.

Differential diagnosis

Rhegmatogenous retinal detachment   The exudative retinal detachments in the V-K-H syndrome are usually bilateral and show the phenomenon of 'shifting fluid' in which the subretinal fluid responds to the force of gravity and detaches the area of the retina under which it accumulates. For example, in the upright position the subretinal

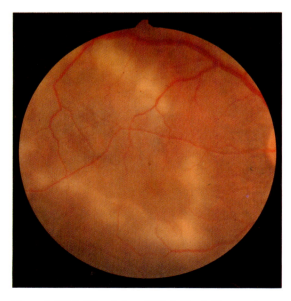

Figure 3.13 Multifocal choroiditis in Vogt–Koyanagi–Harada syndrome (courtesy of Mr E. Glover)

fluid collects inferiorly, but on assuming the supine position the inferior retina flattens and the subretinal fluid shifts posteriorly to detach the macula and superior retina. Exudative retinal detachments are not associated with either retinal breaks or proliferative vitreoretinopathy.

Sympathetic uveitis   Although both conditions cause a bilateral panuveitis and, on occasion, similar systemic features, a history of ocular trauma is absent in V-K-H syndrome and exudative retinal detachment, which is common in V-K-H syndrome, is seldom seen in sympathetic uveitis.

Crohn's disease

Systemic features

Crohn's disease is an idiopathic, chronic, relapsing disease characterized by multifocal granulomas which most frequently involve the terminal ileum and anorectal areas. The disease, which is also frequently referred to as 'granulomatous ileocolitis', 'terminal ileitis', and 'regional ileitis', usually affects young adults. Other parts of the gastrointestinal tract that may also be involved are the oropharynx, oesophagus, stomach, and jejunum. Extraintestinal manifestations include a low-grade fever, weight loss, arthritis, psoriasis, erythema nodosum, and liver disease. The prevalence of HLA-B27 is increased in patients with Crohn's disease, particularly when it is associated with arthritis. About 10% of patients have ocular complications.

Ocular features

Signs

External   Episcleritis is the most common manifestation which may develop with flare-ups of the patient's intestinal symptoms. Some patients also develop a characteristic bilateral, circumferential, peripheral, subepithelial keratopathy. Scleritis is, however, rare.

Slitlamp   Both acute and chronic iridocyclitis may occur. When Crohn's disease is associated with arthritis the incidence of anterior uveitis is increased from 2% to 30%.

Note   Uveitis may, on occasion, precede the occurrence of Crohn's disease.

Vitreous   Cells in the anterior vitreous are seen in patients with iridocyclitis and a more diffuse vitritis is present in eyes with choroiditis.

Fundus   A few patients develop choroiditis or macular oedema.

Note   Patients on long-term intravenous nutrition (hyperalimentation) following bowel resection for Crohn's disease may develop ocular candidiasis (*see* Chapter 7).

Management

Anterior uveitis is treated with topical steroids and choroiditis by systemic steroids. In some patients, surgical resection of diseased intestine results in improvement of intraocular inflammation.

Differential diagnosis

In the past many of the cases described as 'ulcerative colitis' would now, with different criteria, be diagnosed as Crohn's disease. Classically, ulcerative colitis is characterized by diffuse surface ulceration, whereas, in Crohn's disease, the ulceration and inflammation are focal.

Ulcerative colitis

Systemic features

Ulcerative colitis is an idiopathic, chronic, relapsing disease involving the rectum and extending for a variable distance proximally, occasionally to involve the entire colon. The disease is characterized by diffuse surface ulceration of the gut mucosa with the development of crypt abscesses and pseudopolyposis. Extraintestinal manifestations include erythema nodosum, weight loss, anaemia, liver disease, and arthritis (colitic arthritis). Patients with arthritis have an increased

prevalence of HLA-B27 and those with long-standing ulcerative colitis are at increased risk of developing carcinoma of the colon.

Note   Colitic arthritis can be of two types: (1) a mild peripheral arthritis affecting large joints or (2) sacro-iliitis and ankylosing spondylitis.

Ocular features

Signs

External   Episcleritis occurs in some cases.

Slitlamp   Some patients, particularly those with associated sacro-iliitis, develop recurrent attacks of acute anterior uveitis similar to those seen in ankylosing spondylitis. However, unlike the uveitis associated with ankylosing spondylitis, attacks of intraocular inflammation are frequently synchronized with exacerbations of colitis.

Management

The anterior uveitis is treated in the normal way (Chapter 10). In some patients colectomy has a beneficial effect on both the severity and rate of recurrences of intraocular inflammation.

Whipple's disease

Systemic features

Whipple's disease is a very rare multisystem disease characterized by intestinal malabsorption, diarrhoea, abdominal pain, and arthralgia. It typically affects men in the fifth decade of life. Frequently associated systemic features include fever, hypermelanosis, and peripheral lymphadenopathy. Some patients may also have neurological and ocular manifestations. The diagnosis is usually made by jejunal biopsy, which demonstrates the presence of PAS-positive macrophages in the cytoplasm. The ocular manifestations of Whipple's disease result from CNS involvement, direct intraocular inflammation or both.

Ocular features

Signs

External   Ophthalmoplegia, nystagmus and gaze palsy secondary to CNS involvement.

Slitlamp   A chronic iridocyclitis is present in some patients.

Vitreous   Small round white vitreous opacities are occasionally seen.

Fundus   A diffuse chorioretinitis characterized by vasculitis, haemorrhages, exudates, retinal capillary closure, optic disc oedema, and choroidal folds has been described.

Management

Administration of antibiotics is beneficial for both the systemic and ocular manifestations of the disease. Pars plana vitrectomy may have therapeutic as well as diagnostic value.

Further reading

Sarcoidosis

ASDOURIAN, G.K., GOLDBERG, M.F. and BUSSE, B.J. (1975) Peripheral retinal neovascularization in sarcoidosis. *Archives of Ophthalmology*, **93**, 787–790

CAMPO, R.V. and AABERG, T.M. (1984) Choroidal granuloma in sarcoidosis. *Ophthalmology*, **97**, 419–427

CHUMBLEY, L.C. and KEARNS, T.P. (1971) Retinopathy of sarcoidosis. *Transactions of the American Ophthalmological Society*, **69**, 307–310

DOXANAS, M.T., KELLY, J.S. and PROUT, T.E. (1980) Sarcoidosis of the optic nerve head. *American Journal of Ophthalmology*, **90**, 347–351

GASS, D.J.M. and OLSON, C.L. (1976) Sarcoidosis with optic nerve and retinal involvement. *Archives of Ophthalmology*, **94**, 945–948

JAMES, G.D., NEVILLE, E. and LANGLEY, D.S. (1976) Ocular sarcoidosis. *Transactions of the Ophthalmological Society of the United Kingdom*, **96**, 133–139

JAMPOL, L.M., WOODFIN, W. and McLEAN, E.B. (1972) Optic nerve sarcoidosis. *Archives of Ophthalmology*, **87**, 355–360

MARCUS, D.F., BOVINO, J.A. and BURTON, T.C. (1982) Sarcoid granuloma of the choroid. *Ophthalmology*, **89**, 1326–1330

NICHOLSON, C.W., EAGLE, R.C.JR, YANOFF, M. et al. (1980) Conjunctival biopsy as an aid in the evaluation of the patient with suspected sarcoidosis. *Ophthalmology*, **87**, 287–291

OBENAUF, C.D., SHAW, H.E., SYDNOR, C.F. et al. (1978) Sarcoidosis and its ocular manifestations. *American Journal of Ophthalmology*, **86**, 648–655

PERKINS, E.S. (EDITORIAL) (1981) Ocular sarcoidosis. *Archives of Ophthalmology*, **99**, 1193

SANDERS, M.D. and SHILLING, J.S. (1976) Retinal, choroidal and optic disc involvement in sarcoidosis. *Transactions of the Ophthalmological Society of the United Kingdom*, **96**, 140–144

STUDDY, P., BIRD, R. and JAMES, D.G. (1978) Serum angiotensin converting enzyme in sarcoidosis and other granulomatous disorders. *Lancet*, ii, 1331–1334

WEINBERG, R. and TESSLER, H. (1976) Serum lysozyme in sarcoid uveitis. *Ophthalmology*, **82**, 105–108

WEINREB, R.N. (1984) Diagnosing sarcoidosis by transconjunctival biopsy of the lacrimal gland. *American Journal of Ophthalmology*, **97**, 573–576

WEINREB, R.N., BARTH, R. and KIMURA, S.J. (1980) Limited gallium scans and angiotensin converting enzyme in granulomatous uveitis. *Ophthalmology*, **87**, 202–206

WEINREB, R.N. and KIMURA, S.J. (1980) Uveitis associated with sarcoidosis and angiotensin converting enzyme. *American Journal of Ophthalmology*, **89**, 180–185

Behçet's disease

CHAMBERLAIN, M.A. (1978) Behçet's disease. *British Medical Journal*, **2**, 1369–1370

COLLUM, L.M.T., MULLANEY, J. and BOWELL, R. (1981) Current concepts of Behçet's disease. *Transactions of the Ophthalmological Society of the United Kingdom*, **101**, 422–428

COLVARD, D.M., ROBERTSON, D.M. and O'DUFFY, J.D. (1977) The ocular manifestations of Behçet's disease. *Archives of Ophthalmology*, **95**, 1813–1817

JAMES, G.D. and SPITERI, M.A. (1982) Behçet's disease. *Ophthalmology*, **89**, 1279–1284

MAMO, J.G. and AZZAM, S.A. (1970) Treatment of Behçet's disease with chlorambucil. *Archives of Ophthalmology*, **84**, 446–450

O'DUFFY, J.D., ROBERTSON, D.M. and GOLDSTEIN, N.P. (1984) Chlorambucil in the treatment of uveitis and meningoencephalitis of Behçet's disease. *American Journal of Medicine*, **76**, 75–78

OHNO, S. (1981) Immunological aspects of Behçet's and Vogt–Koyanagi–Harada disease. *Transactions of the Ophthalmological Society of the United Kingdom*, **101**, 335–341

PAGE, N.G.R., THOMSON, A. and JAMES, D.G. (1982) Behçet's disease. *Transactions of the Ophthalmological Society of the United Kingdom*, **102**, 174–177

PALIMERIS, G., KOLIOPOULOS, J., THEODOSSIADIS, G. et al. (1980) Adamantiadis–Behçet's syndrome. Clinical and immunological observations. *Transactions of the Ophthalmological Society of the United Kingdom*, **100**, 527–530

Vogt–Koyanagi–Harada syndrome

CARLSON, M.R. and KERMAN, B.M. (1977) Hemorrhagic

macular detachment in the Vogt–Koyanagi–Harada syndrome. *American Journal of Ophthalmology*, **84**, 632–635

OHNO, S., CHAR, D.H., KIMURA, S.J. *et al.* (1977) Vogt–Koyanagi–Harada syndrome. *American Journal of Ophthalmology*, **83**, 735–740

SNYDER, D.A. and TESSLER, H. (1980) Vogt–Koyanagi–Harada syndrome. *American Journal of Ophthalmology*, **90**, 69–73

Crohn's disease

HOPKINS, D.J., HORAN, E., BURTON, I.L. *et al.* (1974) Ocular disorders in a series of 332 patients with Crohn's disease. *British Journal of Ophthalmology*, **58**, 732–737

KNOX, D.L., SCHACHAT, A.P. and MUSTONEN, E. (1984) Primary, secondary and coincidental ocular complications of Crohn's disease. *Ophthalmology*, **91**, 163–173

KNOX, D.L., SNIP, R.C. and STARK, W.J. (1980) The keratopathy of Crohn's disease. *American Journal of Ophthalmology*, **90**, 862–865

MACOUL, K.L. (1970) Ocular changes in granulomatous ileocolitis. *Archives of Ophthalmology*, **84**, 95–97

Ulcerative colitis

KORELITZ, B.I. and COLES, R.S. (1967) Uveitis (iritis) associated with ulcerative colitis and granulomatous colitis. *Gastroenterology*, **52**, 78–82

Whipple's disease

AVILA, M.P., JALKH, A.E., FELDMAN, E. *et al.* (1984) Manifestations of Whipple's disease in the posterior segment of the eye. *Archives of Ophthalmology*, **102**, 384–390

FONT, R.L., RAO, N.A., ISSARESCU, S. *et al.* (1978) Ocular involvement in Whipple's disease. *Archives of Ophthalmology*, **96**, 1431–1436

4

Chronic systemic infections

Acquired syphilis

Syphilis is a chronic infection caused by a spirochaete called *Treponema pallidum*. The disease may be acquired or congenital.

Systemic features

Acquired syphilis is a venereal infection which can be divided into four stages.

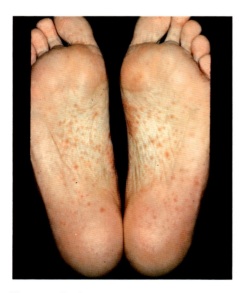

Figure 4.1 Rash in secondary syphilis (courtesy of Dr J. Haynes)

Primary This stage occurs between 10 days and 10 weeks following sexual contact. It is characterized by a painless indurated ulcer (chancre) usually located on the genitalia.

Secondary The hallmark of secondary syphilis, which usually develops between three and six weeks after the chancre, is the appearance of a macular, papular, or mixed skin rash involving the palms and soles (*Figure 4.1*). Other features include malaise, fever, generalized lymphadenopathy, condylomata lata, mucous patches and meningitis.

Latent This follows resolution of secondary syphilis and can be detected only by serological tests.

Tertiary About 15% of patients with untreated latent syphilis eventually develop tertiary syphilis, although many patients have tertiary syphilis without definite preceding manifestations of the primary and secondary stages. The four types of tertiary syphilis are: meningovascular, tabes dorsalis, general paralysis of the insane (GPI), and gummatous.

Diagnostic tests

FTA-ABS (fluorescent treponemal antibody absorption) This is a specific test to detect anti-treponemal antibodies. Once positive the test will remain positive throughout the patient's life despite treatment. However, the test is not titratable and is read as: reactive, weakly reactive, or non-reactive.

VDRL (Venereal Disease Research Laboratory)
This is a non-specific reagin test which is useful for screening. It becomes positive shortly after the development of the primary chancre. The test is titratable, but it may become negative after many years in about 40% of patients. It also frequently becomes negative following adequate anti-syphilitic therapy.

> *Note* If syphilis is suspected as a cause of uveitis, both tests should be ordered. The FTA-ABS, because of its high specificity and sensitivity, and the VDRL to determine the degree of disease activity.

Ocular features

Syphilis is now a relatively rare cause of uveitis accounting for about 1% of cases. The disease must be suspected in any case of intraocular inflammation that is resistant to treatment with conventional therapy.

Signs

External A primary chancre may, very occasionally, occur in the conjunctiva. The patient may also have loss of eyebrows and eyelashes (madarosis).

Slitlamp An iridocyclitis occurs in about 4% of patients with secondary syphilis. The intraocular inflammation is usually acute and it may be granulomatous or non-granulomatous and, unless adequately treated, it becomes chronic. Both eyes are involved in about 50% of cases. In some patients, the iridocyclitis is first associated with the presence of roseolae (*Figure 4.2*) which consist of hyperaemic bright-red spots representing engorged pre-existing superficial vascular loops of the iris. The roseolae may then develop into more localized papules and subsequently into larger well-defined yellowish nodules. Gummas, which are characteristically located at the root of the iris, are extremely rare.

Vitreous The vitreous is involved in eyes with posterior uveitis.

Fundus Syphilis can involve the choroid and retina.

Chorioretinitis, which is bilateral in about 50% of cases, is usually either multifocal or diffuse. The former is non-specific but the latter is characterized by a diffuse greyish-yellow exudation which may be most marked in the mid-retinal periphery and may surround the optic disc. A periarteritis and periphlebitis, similar to that seen in sarcoidosis, may also be present.

Neuroretinitis consists of primary involvement of the retina and optic nerve head and is independent of choroidal inflammation. It occurs usually during secondary syphilis and it may be associated with meningitis. The fundus shows a greyish clouding of the retina due to oedema, most marked at the posterior pole. The optic disc is elevated and its margins indistinct. The retinal veins may be engorged and peripapillary cotton-wool spots or flame-shaped haemorrhages may appear, as well as perimacular waxy exudates.

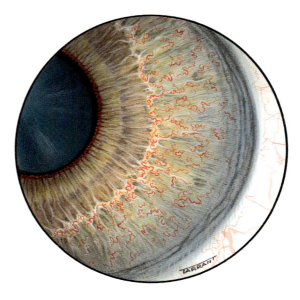

Figure 4.2 Early roseolae in secondary syphilis

Clinical course and complications

Chorioretinitis   Unless adequately treated, the intraocular inflammation runs a protracted course. Its healed stage is occasionally characterized by extensive pigmentary changes with perivascular bone spicules similar to those seen in retinitis pigmentosa. These changes may be associated with night blindness and a ring scotoma.

Neuroretinitis   Unless treated with anti-syphilitic drugs the disease progresses and the retinal vessels are replaced by white strands, the optic disc becomes atrophic, and areas of hyperpigmentation develop (*Figure 4.3*).

Management

Treatment of syphilitic uveitis is as follows: the patient should be hospitalized and a lumbar puncture performed to rule out neurosyphilis. The following antibiotics should be administered if the patient is not sensitive to penicillin.

1 Aqueous crystalline penicillin G, $2–4 \times 10^6$ units intravenously every 4 h for 10 days.
2 Aqueous penicillin G procaine, 2.4×10^6 units intramuscularly daily for 10 days.

Oral probenecid 500 mg every 6 h for 10 days should also be administered to elevate and prolong the plasma level of penicillin. Patients who are allergic to penicillin can be treated with oral erythromycin 500 mg four times a day for 15 days.

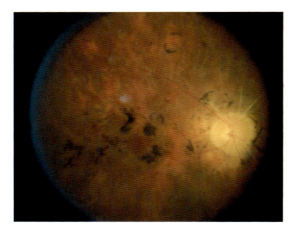

Figure 4.3 End-stage syphilitic neuroretinitis

Congenital syphilis

Systemic features

The classical Hutchinson's triad of congenital syphilis consists of interstitial keratitis, deafness and typical changes of the teeth. Other stigmata include rhagades, sabre shin, saddle nose, and Clutton's joints.

Ocular features

Signs

External   Interstitial keratitis is a late manifestation of congenital syphilis which usually develops between the ages of 5 and 25 years. It is characterized by a bilateral acute diffuse keratitis which causes severe visual impairment. Deep neovascularization then develops and, when the new vessels meet in the centre of the cornea, they give rise to the so-called 'salmon patch'. After a few months the cornea begins to clear and the vessels become non-perfused (ghost vessels). If the eye becomes inflamed again the vessels may refill with blood.

Slitlamp   An anterior uveitis is always present in eyes with acute interstitial keratitis.

Fundus   This may show a finely pigmented peripheral 'salt and pepper' appearance which is non-progressive and benign.

Management

Treatment of acute interstitial keratitis is with topical steroids.

Tuberculosis

Systemic features

Tuberculosis (TB) is a chronic granulomatous infection caused by either bovine or human tubercle bacilli. The former causes TB by the drinking of milk from infected cattle and the latter is spread by 'droplet infection'. The two main forms of TB are primary and post-primary.

Primary TB

This occurs in subjects not previously exposed to the bacillus. It typically causes the 'primary complex' in the chest (Ghon focus + regional lymphadenopathy) which usually heals spontaneously and causes little if any systemic symptoms.

Post-primary TB

This is due to reinfection or, rarely, recrudescence of a primary lesion, usually in a patient with impaired immunity as from diabetes, systemic steroid therapy, or malnutrition. Clinical features of post-primary TB include fibrocaseous pulmonary lesions, and miliary TB from haematogenous spread to many parts of the body. Theoretically, uveal seeding by live bacilli may occur during the primary and miliary stages giving rise to either caseating nodules or small miliary tubercles.

Diagnostic tests

Examination of sputum　This is for acid-fast bacilli.

Chest X-ray　A chest X-ray compatible with TB is of significance in a patient with uveitis. However, a negative chest X-ray does not necessarily exclude the possibility of TB.

Tuberculin test　This may be useful in the diagnosis of extrathoracic TB. In the United Kingdom, less than 4% of English-born children have a positive test when tested at the age of 12 years. However, no importance can be attached to a positive result in a subject who has either received BCG or who has had TB in the past. A negative test usually excludes the possibility of TB whereas a positive test does not necessarily distinguish between previous exposure and active disease.

Isoniazid test　If TB uveitis is suspected, a therapeutic test of isoniazid 300 mg daily for three weeks has been recommended. If this causes a dramatic improvement in the ocular inflammation within one or two weeks then the diagnosis of TB is highly likely.

Ocular features

TB is now a rare cause of uveitis accounting for only about 1% of all cases. Despite this it is important not to miss the diagnosis as it is one of the few causes of uveal inflammation which can be cured with specific medication. The possibility of TB is always presumptive and is based on indirect evidence, such as: intractable uveitis which is unresponsive to steroid therapy, negative findings for other causes of uveitis, positive systemic findings for TB and, occasionally, a positive response to the isoniazid test.

Signs

There is no specific finding in TB uveitis and the clinical picture is pleomorphic.

External　Virtually any ocular and periocular structure can be involved including the orbit, skin, conjunctiva and cornea.

Slitlamp　The most common finding is a chronic granulomatous iridocyclitis although occasionally the inflammation is non-granulomatous.

Vitreous　In eyes with choroiditis, vitreous involvement is usually mild.

Fundus　TB primarily involves the choroid. The most frequent finding is a focal (*see Figure 1.16*) or multifocal choroiditis. Rarely, a large solitary choroidal granuloma, which may be mistaken for a choroidal tumour, may be present in one eye of a patient with chronic pulmonary TB.

Management

Treatment is with isoniazid 300 mg/day and 10 mg/day of pyridoxine hydrochloride (to prevent peripheral neuritis) combined with one other anti-tuberculous drug such as rifampicin for 12 months. Ocular penetration of izoniazid is very good although some patients become intolerant.

Leprosy

Systemic features

Leprosy (Hansen's disease) has the highest incidence of ocular complications of any systemic disease. The pathogenic agent responsible for leprosy is *Mycobacterium leprae* which has an affinity for skin, peripheral nerves and the anterior segment of the eye. The two types are lepromatous and tuberculoid leprosy. Uveal involvement in tuberculoid disease is less common than in the lepromatous form.

Ocular features

Signs

External The many lesions of the anterior segment include madarosis, keratitis (due to a combination of trichiasis, lagophthalmos, loss of corneal sensation, and secondary infection), conjunctivitis, scleritis, and episcleritis.

Slitlamp The complications of anterior uveitis are the most common causes of blindness in leprosy. The uveitis can be of two types:

Acute iritis is thought to be caused by the deposition of immune complexes in the anterior uvea and it may be associated with systemic symptoms such as fever and swelling of skin lesions. Occasionally the intraocular inflammation is precipitated by the initiation or withdrawal of anti-lepromatous systemic therapy.

Chronic iritis is due to direct invasion of the anterior uvea by bacilli. A relatively common finding is the presence at the pupillary margin of small glistening 'iris pearls' which resemble a necklace (*Figure 4.4a*). These lesions, which are composed of bacilli within histiocytes, are pathognomonic of lepromatous leprosy. The 'pearls' slowly enlarge and coalesce before becoming pedunculated and dropping into the anterior chamber (*Figure 4.4b*) from which they eventually disappear. Much less common than 'iris pearls' are nodular lepromata which are yellow, globular, polymorphic, single masses which, just like 'iris pearls', may be seen in uninflamed eyes. Eventually the iris becomes atrophic and the associated formation of holes in the iris stroma may give rise to an appearance similar to essential iris atrophy.

Note Miosis is frequently present in eyes with chronic iritis and this, combined with secondary cataract and corneal opacification, is a major cause of visual impairment.

Fundus This is not involved.

Management

Acute anterior uveitis is treated with topical mydriatics and steroids. By contrast the chronic form is more resistant to conventional therapy. It is thought that this is because it is not a true inflammation, but rather a form of neuroparalytic uveitis caused by early involvement of the iris nerves. Eyes with chronic uveitis usually tolerate surgery for secondary cataracts very well.

Further reading

Syphilis
ARRUGA, J., VALENTINES, J., MAURI, F. *et al.* (1985) Neuroretinitis in acquired syphilis. *Ophthalmology*, **92**, 262–270
BELIN, M.W., BALTCH, A.L. and HAY, P.B. (1981) Secondary syphilitic uveitis. *American Journal of Ophthalmology*, **92**, 210–214

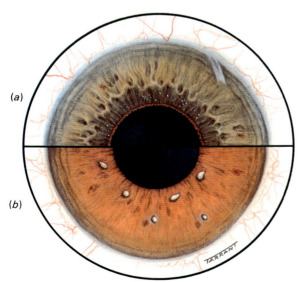

(a)

(b)

Figure 4.4 Chronic lepromatous iridocyclitis. (a) Small 'iris pearls', (b) large 'iris pearls' some of which have dropped into the anterior chamber

FOLK, J.C., WEINGEIST, T.A., CORBETT, J.J. *et al.* (1983) Syphilitic neuroretinitis. *American Journal of Ophthalmology*, **95**, 480–486

ROSS, W.H. and SUTTON, H.F.S. (1980) Acquired syphilitic uveitis. *Archives of Ophthalmology*, **98**, 496–498

SCHLAEGEL, T.F. JR and KAO, S.F. (1982) A review (1970–1980) of 28 presumptive cases of syphilitic uveitis. *American Journal of Ophthalmology*, **93**, 412–414

SCHWARTZ, L.K. and O'CONNOR, G.R. (1980) Secondary syphilis with iris papules. *American Journal of Ophthalmology*, **90**, 380–384

ZWINK, F.B. and DUNLOP, E.M.C. (1976) Clinically silent anterior uveitis in secondary syphilis. *Transactions of the Ophthalmological Society of the United Kingdom*, **96**, 148–150

Tuberculosis

ABRAMS, J. and SCHLAEGEL, T.F.JR (1982) The role of the Isoniazid therapeutic test in tuberculous uveitis. *American Journal of Ophthalmology*, **94**, 511–515

JABBOUR, N.M., FARIS, B. and TREMPE, C.L. (1985) A case of tuberculosis presenting with choroidal tuberculoma. *Ophthalmology*, **92**, 834–837

SCHLAEGEL, T.F.JR (1981) Bacterial and protozoal uveitis. *Transactions of the Ophthalmological Society of the United Kingdom*, **101**, 312–316

Leprosy

FFYTCHE, T.J. (1981) Iritis in leprosy. *Transactions of the Ophthalmological Society of the United Kingdom*, **101**, 325–327

FFYTCHE, T.J. (1981) Role of iris changes as a cause of blindness in lepromatous leprosy. *British Journal of Ophthalmology*, **65**, 231–239

FFYTCHE, T.J. (1981) Cataract surgery in the management of the late complications of lepromatous leprosy in South Korea. *British Journal of Ophthalmology*, **65**, 243–248

MICHELSON, J.B., ROTH, A.M. and WARING, G.O. (1979) Lepromatous iridocyclitis diagnosed by anterior chamber paracentesis. *American Journal of Ophthalmology*, **88**, 674–679

SPAIDE, R., NATTIS, R., LIPKA, A. *et al.* (1985) Ocular findings in leprosy in the United States. *American Journal of Ophthalmology*, **100**, 411–416

5

Parasitic infestations

Toxoplasmosis

Introduction

Toxoplasmosis is an infestation by a ubiquitous, obligatory, intracellular protozoan parasite *Toxoplasma gondii*. The cat is the definitive host of the parasite and other animals, such as mice and livestock (cattle, sheep and pigs), as well as humans, are intermediate hosts.

Forms of Toxoplasma gondii

The three main forms of the parasite are:

1 The *oocyst* is the spore form which is excreted in cat faeces.
2 The *bradyzoite* is the inactive slowly metabolizing form which is encysted in tissues.
3 The *tachyzoite* (trophozoite) is the proliferating active form which is responsible for tissue destruction and inflammation. It has a particular affinity for neural tissue and causes acute retinitis in humans.

Modes of infestation of humans

Humans can become infested by toxoplasmosis in three main ways.

Ingestion of undercooked meat It is thought that the most common mode of infestation is by the ingestion of raw meat such as steak tartare or undercooked hamburgers. In this way humans acquire toxoplasmosis by eating the flesh of an intermediate host which contains tissue cysts.

Ingestion of oocysts This is probably a less common way of human infestation although it is the primary mode of infestation of animal intermediate hosts. Humans may accidentally contaminate their hands when disposing of cat litter trays and then transfer the oocysts onto food. Small children may also become infested by eating dirt (pica) containing oocysts. The oocyst may also be transferred to food by vectors such as flies.

Transplacental If a pregnant woman develops acute toxoplasmosis, the parasites (tachyzoites) may pass through the placenta to infest the fetus.

Three stages of toxoplasmosis

In humans, toxoplasmosis can be divided into three stages:

1 *Acute* When ingested by humans, the parasites penetrate the intestinal mucosa, gain access to the blood stream and become disseminated throughout the body. They then enter the cells of the reticuloendothelial system, the brain, the retina, the lungs and striated muscles where they rapidly multiply and cause the acute form of the disease (which is usually asymptomatic). At this stage the host defence mechanism reacts to the parasite and specific anti-toxoplasma antibodies are produced.

2 *Chronic (inactive)* When the acute proliferative phase of toxoplasmosis is curtailed, the parasites form intracellular cysts which contain slowly metabolizing inactive parasites (bradyzoites).

> *Note* These 'tissue' cysts may lie dormant in the neuroretina throughout the patient's life with no ill-effects.

3 Recurrent In some cases the patient's immune mechanism is suppressed, the cyst walls rupture, releasing active and prolifertaing parasites (tachyzoites) which invade and destroy healthy cells, causing recurrence of the disease.

> *Note* The vast majority of ocular toxoplasmosis is due to recurrences.

Diagnostic tests

Dye test (Sabin–Feldman)

This test is based on the fact that live organisms exposed to normal serum take up methylene blue, whereas those exposed to serum containing anti-toxoplasma antibodies fail to take up the dye.

Indirect fluorescent antibody (IFA) test

This test utilizes killed organisms which are exposed to the patient's serum and anti-human globulin labelled with fluorescein and examined under the fluorescent microscope.

Haemagglutination test

In this test, lysed organisms are coated onto red blood cells which are then exposed to the patient's serum. Positive sera cause the red blood cells to agglutinate.

Enzyme-linked immunosorbant assay (ELISA)

In this test the patient's antibodies bind to an excess of solid-phase antigen. This complex is then incubated with an enzyme-linked second antibody. Assessment of enzyme activity provides the measurement of specific antibody concentration. The test can also be used to detect antibodies in the aqueous humour and the vitreous.

> *Note*
> 1 The ELISA technique can also be applied to the serodiagnosis of toxocariasis.
> 2 Although the Sabin–Feldman dye test is extremely accurate it requires the maintenance of live *Toxoplasma gondii* and consequently has been rejected by many laboratories. The IFA and ELISA are now the two most frequently used tests and are essentially similar in sensitivity and specificity.
> 3 It should be emphasized that ocular toxoplasmosis may not elevate the titres of the serological tests. Therefore, any positive result, even in undiluted serum (1:1) is significant. The ophthalmologist should therefore ensure that the laboratory report any titre, even on an undiluted specimen. Since about 50% of the general population have positive serology, a positive result does not necessarily mean that the ocular inflammation is caused by toxoplasmosis. However, if the serological tests are negative, even with undiluted serum, it is very unlikely that the patient's intraocular inflammation is caused by toxoplasmosis.

Acute acquired systemic toxoplasmosis

Clinical features

The infestation may present in the following ways.

Subclinical

The vast majority of patients are completely asymptomatic when they acquire the infestation.

Febrile lymphadenitis

In some patients the disease causes a generalized lymphadenopathy, malaise, and headaches. This 'lymphadenopathic' form resembles glandular fever and persists for about four weeks.

'Influenza-like'

In a few patients, the acute infestation resembles influenza and is characterized by malaise, headache, inertia, fever, and muscle aching which lasts for about 10 days.

Meningoencephalitis

Very occasionally, acute toxoplasmosis gives rise to convulsions, unconsciousness, fever, and lymphadenopathy.

Exanthematous form

By far the rarest and most serious form of acute toxoplasmosis, which may be fatal, resembles a rickettsial infection and is characterized by fever, chills, a macular rash, and cough.

> *Note* Only about 2% of patients with acute acquired toxoplasmosis have ocular involvement. In contrast to the congenital form (which will be described later), acquired lesions are not associated with old scars in either eye.

Congenital systemic toxoplasmosis

Clinical features

Toxoplasmosis is transmitted to the fetus through the placenta when a pregnant woman contracts the acute infestation (which is usually asymptomatic). If the mother is infested before pregnancy the fetus will not be affected. About 40% of infants born to recently infested mothers will acquire toxoplasmosis which may be inactive or active at the time of birth.

Active at birth

The severity of involvement of the fetus varies with the duration of gestation at the time of maternal infestation.

Death If the infestation is acquired during early pregnancy the fetus may be stillborn.

Severe damage or miscarriage If the infestation is acquired in midpregnancy, the fetus may be spontaneously aborted or it may have severe brain damage in the form of hydrocephalus or microcephalus.

Convulsions If the infestation is acquired during late pregnancy, the fetus may suffer from generalised convulsions, paralysis, fever, visceral involvement and chorioretinitis. Skull X-rays may show intracranial calcification (*Figure 5.1*).

> *Note* The 'three Cs' of congenital toxoplasmosis are convulsions, chorioretinitis, and calcification.

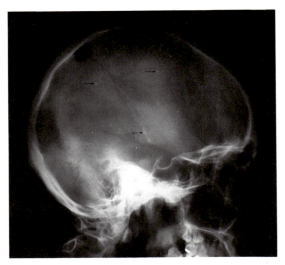

Figure 5.1 Intracranial calcification in congenital toxoplasmosis (courtesy of Dr I. Yentis)

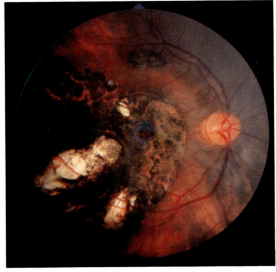

Figure 5.2 Healed toxoplasma retinochoroiditis

Inactive at birth

Just as in the acquired form, most cases of congenital systemic toxoplasmosis are subclinical. In these children, bilateral healed chorioretinal scars (*Figure 5.2*) may be discovered later in life either by chance on a routine fundus examination or when the child is found to have defective vision.

> *Note* In the past, these macular scars were frequently incorrectly termed 'macular colobomas'.

Recurrent toxoplasmic retinochoroiditis

Recurrence of old healed congenital ocular toxoplasmosis is responsible for between 50% and 75% of all cases of posterior uveitis in the United States and the United Kingdom. The recurrences usually take place between the ages of 10 and 35 years (average age is 25 years) when the cysts rupture and release hundreds of parasites (tachyzoites) into normal retinal cells.

> *Note* The primary lesion is a retinitis and the inflammatory reaction seen in the choroid, iris, and retinal blood vessels is believed to be immune in origin and not actually due to direct infestation.

Clinical features

Symptoms

Depending on the site of the lesion, the symptoms are floaters and blurred vision.

Signs

External The eye is usually white.

Slitlamp The anterior chamber may be quiet or it may occasionally show a non-granulomatous or granulomatous iridocyclitis.

> *Note* A fundus examination through a dilated pupil should be performed on all patients presenting with an anterior uveitis to eliminate the possibility of an underlying posterior uveitis.

Vitreous The retinitis is usually accompanied by a severe vitritis which can frequently be traced back to the inflammatory focus. The posterior vitreous may become detached and the posterior hyaloid face covered by inflammatory precipitates comparable to keratic precipitates. In severe cases the vitritis may preclude visualization of the fundus with the direct ophthalmoscope.

Fundus Fundus lesions are of several types:

Focal necrotizing retinitis, adjacent to the edge of an old inactive pigmented scar ('satellite lesion'), is by far the most common finding. The lesion is most commonly solitary although multifocal retinitis may also occur and occasionally the lesion develops in an area of the retina that appears ophthalmoscopically normal. Although all parts of the fundus are at risk, the retinitis typically affects the post-equatorial fundus. Active retinitis is characterized by a white or yellow-white lesion with fluffy indistinct edges (*Figure 5.3*). It may vary in size from one-tenth to five disc diameters

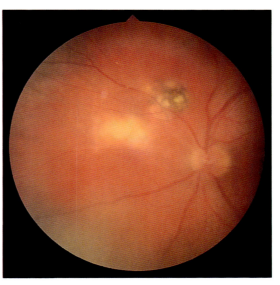

Figure 5.3 Active toxoplasma retinochoroiditis

and is associated with an overlying vitreous haze and vitreous condensation. The active lesion may be associated with an arteritis which characteristically involves the artery leading to the lesion. A periphlebitis may also be seen at the site of the retinitis or in remote areas of the fundus. Very occasionally the vasculitis causes arteriolar obstruction or a branch vein occlusion. In some cases yellow, lipid-like, refractile plaques are present along the major branch arteries.

> *Note* Active bilateral toxoplasma retinitis is extremely rare, although old scars are usually seen in both eyes.

Deep retinitis is much less common than the superficial retinitis just described. Here the inflammatory focus is located in the deeper retinal layers and appears yellow, has more distinct borders and is not associated with an overlying vitritis. In some cases the deep focus evolves into the more typical lesion within one or two weeks.

Punctate outer retinal toxoplasmosis is very rare. It is characterized by multifocal punctate outer retinal lesions with little or no vitreous involvement. The lesions are at the level of the deep retina and retinal pigment epithelium, and appear grey-white in colour. They resolve slowly and recur in a satellite fashion in adjacent areas.

> *Note* Deep toxoplasma retinitis may lead to diagnostic difficulties unless old toxoplasma scars are also present.

Massive granuloma is another rare finding characterized by lesions that are greater than six disc diameters in size with sharply defined borders and amorphous centres. The granuloma may be difficult to visualize because of extensive involvement of the vitreous.

Papillitis—not infrequently the active retinitis is located in the juxtapapillary area (Jensen's choroiditis) and occasionally the optic nerve head itself is the primary site of involvement. The papillitis is characterized by a white inflammatory mass on the optic disc with an overlying vitreous haze.

Visual acuity is usually relatively good unless the macula or the papillomacular bundle is also involved.

Clinical course and complications

The rate of healing is dependent on the virulence of the organism, the competence of the host's immune system, and the use of antimicrobial drugs. In uncompromised hosts the retinitis heals within 1–4 months and is replaced by a sharply demarcated atrophic scar surrounded by a hyperpigmented border. The vitreous haze gradually clears although vitreous condensation may remain. Resolution of anterior uveitis is a reliable sign of posterior segment healing. In a small percentage of cases, the intraocular inflammation persists for up to two years despite intensive antimicrobial and steroid therapy. Fulmination inflammation occurs most commonly when the retinitis is treated with steroids alone or in immunosuppressed patients. After the first attack, the rate of further recurrences is 2.7 per patient.

Eyes with toxoplasmosis may lose vision from various direct or indirect causes.

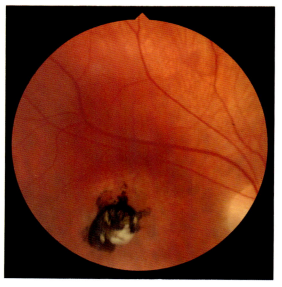

Figure 5.4 Healed toxoplasma retinochoroiditis involving fovea

Direct

1 Involvement of the fovea (*Figure 5.4*).
2 Involvement of the papillomacular bundle.
3 Involvement of the optic nerve head (rare).

Indirect

1 Cystoid macular oedema from an extrafoveal lesion (*Figure 5.5*).
2 Macular pucker with wrinkling of the fovea may occur in some eyes in which the fovea is not directly involved.
3 Subretinal neovascularization leading to subretinal haemorrhage has been reported.
4 Retinal neovascularization which may lead to secondary vitreous haemorrhage, is a very rare sequel to the inactive phase.
5 Tractional retinal detachment due to extensive vitreous fibrosis is also rare.

Note This complication may respond to treatment by pars plana vitrectomy.

---

6 Rhegmatogenous retinal detachment due to breaks occurring during active retinitis.

Management

Indications

It is important to realize that not all active lesions need treatment because small peripheral foci may be self-limiting and relatively innocuous (*Figure 5.6*). There are three main indications for medical therapy of active toxoplasma retinitis.

1 A lesion involving or threatening the macula or the papillomacular bundle.
2 A lesion threatening or involving the optic nerve head.
3 A very severe vitritis that has caused severe visual impairment and which subsequently may be responsible for vitreous fibrosis and tractional retinal detachment.

Unless at least one of these criteria apply, treatment is unnecessary because the drugs currently available may have serious side-effects. The following drugs are used in the treatment of toxoplasma retinitis.

Steroids
1 Topical steroids are useful in the management of associated anterior uveitis but they have no effect on posterior segment inflammation.

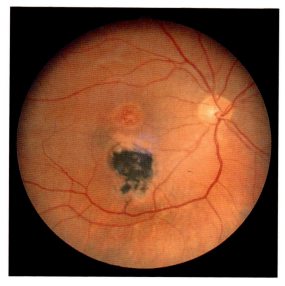

Figure 5.5 Macular hole due to chronic cystoid macular oedema adjacent to a toxoplasma scar

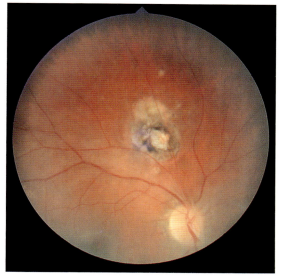

Figure 5.6 Small 'satellite' active lesion not requiring treatment

2 Periocular steroid injections—anterior sub-Tenon's injection can be used to treat severe anterior uveitis and some authorities recommend the use of posterior sub-Tenon's injection in preference to systemic steroids for posterior segment inflammation.

3 Systemic therapy is recommended in eyes with vision-threatening lesions, particularly if associated with severe vitritis.

Note
a The rationale for using steroids is to counteract immunologically induced retinal damage.
b Steroids may compromise the patient's immune system and exacerbate the ocular inflammation.
c Steroids should always be used in combination with antimicrobials.

Antimicrobial drugs   The three drugs currently most widely used in the treatment of ocular toxoplasmosis are clindamycin, sulphonamides and pyrimethamine. Because of its toxicity, pyrimethamine is usually now considered as the third drug of choice in patients unresponsive to clindamycin and sulphonamides.

Note   Antimicrobial therapy is of no value in the treatment of inactive disease because the drugs cannot penetrate the cysts that lie dormant in the retina.

Clindamycin   is given orally 300 mg four times a day for three weeks. However, if used alone it may cause a pseudomembranous colitis in some patients so that the patient should be advised to report any persistent cramps and diarrhoea immediately. Treatment of colitis is with oral vancomycin 500 mg every 6 hours for 10 days. The risk of colitis seems to be very much reduced when clindamycin is used together with sulphonamides, as the latter appears to inhibit clostridial overgrowth which is responsible for the colitis.

Sulphonamides   either in the form of sulphadiazine or the mixed sulphonamide Sulphatriad (if available). A loading dose of 2 g is given orally followed by 1 g four times a day for 3–4 weeks. Rare side-effects of sulphonamides are renal stones and allergic reactions. The Stevens–Johnson syndrome is, very occasionally, triggered off by these drugs.

Pyrimethamine   (Daraprim) is a folic acid antagonist which may cause thrombocytopenia and leucopenia. For this reason weekly blood counts should be performed and the drug used only in combination with folinic acid 10 mg/day orally (mixed with orange juice) as this counteracts the toxic side-effects of folic acid antagonists. The loading dose of pyrimethamine is 75–150 mg followed by 25 mg daily for 3–4 weeks. Only a one-week course should be given if it is combined with clindamycin.

Differential diagnosis

Candidiasis

The early superficial retinal granuloma of candidiasis may initially resemble toxoplasma retinitis. However, the lesion is not associated with a healed chorioretinal scar and, as it enlarges, it first bulges into, and then floats in, the vitreous cavity (*see* Chapter 7).

Toxocariasis

The healed posterior pole granuloma of toxocariasis is usually elevated above the retinal surface and is not associated with a healed chorioretinal scar (*Figure 5.7*).

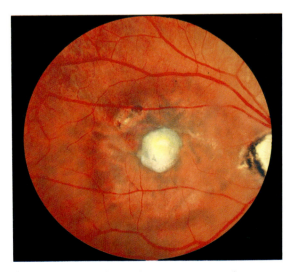

Figure 5.7 Toxocaral granuloma at posterior pole (courtesy of Mr C. Migdal)

Presumed ocular histoplasmosis (POH)

The inactive scars of POH resemble those of toxoplasmosis except that they are usually smaller and are often associated with peripapillary atrophy. The vitreous in POH is normal without signs of previous vitritis (*see* Chapter 7).

Toxocariasis

Introduction

Toxocariasis is an infestation caused by a common intestinal roundworm of cats (*Toxocara cati*) and dogs (*Toxocara canis*). Human infestation is due to accidental ingestion of soil or food contaminated with ova which are shed in dog's faeces. Young children who eat dirt (pica) or are in close contact with puppies are at particular risk of acquiring the disease. Surveys have shown that the prevalence of infestation in puppies two to six months of age is greater than 80%. In the human intestine, the ova develop into larvae which penetrate the intestinal wall and travel to various organs such as the liver, lungs, skin, brain and eyes. When the larva die they disintegrate and cause an inflammatory reaction followed by granulation. Clinically, human infestation can take one of two forms, visceral larva migrans and ocular toxocariasis.

> *Note* Although *Toxocara cati* has been recovered from the human bowel, it has never been found in the eye.

Visceral larval migrans

Visceral larva migrans (VLM) is due to severe systemic infestation which usually occurs at about the age of two years. It is characterized by a low-grade fever, hepatosplenomegaly, pneumonitis which causes wheezing, and convulsions if the brain is involved. The patient's blood film shows a leucocytosis and a marked eosinophilia. The severity of VLM varies from patient to patient and those with very severe infestation may die.

> *Note* Patients with VLM virtually never have ocular involvement.

Diagnostic tests

The ELISA (enzyme-linked immunosorbant assay) test is very useful in identifying patients with toxocariasis as it is highly sensitive and specific. Although, at present, a dilution of 1:8 is considered positive, recent evidence suggests that the presence of any antibody (even in undiluted serum) may be significant.

Ocular toxocariasis

The clinical syndrome of ocular toxocariasis differs markedly from VLM. The patients are otherwise healthy and they have a normal white cell count with absence of eosinophilia. A history of pica is less common, and the average age of patients with ocular involvement is considerably older (7.5 years) as compared with VLM (2 years). The three most common ocular lesions are: a chronic endophthalmitis-like picture, a peripheral granuloma, and a posterior pole granuloma. Other less common manifestations include: a pars planitis-like syndrome, anterior uveitis with or without hypopyon, optic papillitis, localized vitreous abscess and retinal tracks. Only the three most common lesions, all of which are unilateral, will be described in detail.

Chronic endophthalmitis

This usually presents between the ages of two and nine years with leukocoria, strabismus, or a unilateral loss of vision.

Signs

External The eye is usually white although occasionally it is slightly injected.

Slitlamp A mild anterior uveitis is common but the cells and flare are rarely more than +2. Posterior synechiae may develop in severe cases.

Vitreous   Diffusely infiltrated with inflammatory cells and debris.

Fundus   A peripheral granuloma may be seen in some eyes. In other cases the peripheral retina and pars plana is covered by a dense greyish-white exudate similar to the 'snowbanking' seen in pars planitis (*see Figure 8.3*).

Clinical course and complications

The visual prognosis is very poor and some eyes eventually require enucleation. The main causes of visual impairment are:

Retinal detachment   The vitritis may result in the formation of vitreoretinal membranes which, on contraction, may cause either tractional or rhegmatogenous retinal detachments.

Cyclitic membranes   In severe cases, retrolental cyclitic membranes form and, by circumferential traction, pull the ciliary body away from the sclera causing ocular hypotony and, eventually, phthisis bulbi.

Macular oedema   may be present in some eyes.

Cataract

Differential diagnosis

Retinoblastoma   The leukocoria caused by a cyclitic membrane or a large retinal detachment may be mistaken for a retinoblastoma. However, retinoblastoma usually occurs in younger children and may at times be bilateral, whereas ocular toxocariasis is always unilateral. Calcification is a feature of retinoblastoma but not of ocular toxocariasis.

Pars planitis   The 'snowbanking' and vitritis may be similar to that seen in pars planitis. Although pars planitis also occurs in children of the same age group, it is usually bilateral.

Coats' disease   Just like ocular toxoplasmosis, Coats' disease typically affects one eye of a young individual and in severe cases it may be associated with exudative retinal detachment, leukocoria, cataract, and uveitis. However, the marked subretinal yellow exudation and retinal telangiectasia, which is typical of Coats' disease, seldom occurs in ocular toxocariasis.

Posterior pole granuloma

This usually presents between the ages of six and 14 years with unilateral loss of vision.

Signs

External   The eye is invariably white.

Slitlamp   The anterior chamber is quiet.

Vitreous   A few cells may overlie the lesion.

Fundus   The granuloma is round, solitary and located either at the macula (*see Figure 5.7*) or between the macula and the optic disc. The lesion has a yellow-white colour, is slightly elevated above the retinal surface and is usually between one and two disc diameters in size. Retinal stress lines and distortion of the retinal vasculature are frequent associated findings and occasionally retinal blood vessels disappear into the umbilicated lesion. Occasionally, the granuloma is surrounded by hard yellow exudates.

Clinical course and complications

Once formed, the granuloma is usually stationary and the extent of visual loss is dependent on its location. Rare complications include serous retinal detachment and subretinal haemorrhage.

Differential diagnosis

Toxoplasmosis   The scars of healed toxoplasma retinochoroiditis are usually flat, associated with hyperpigmentation (*see Figure 5.5*) and frequently bilateral.

Peripheral granuloma

This usually presents between the ages of six and 40 years. In uncomplicated cases, visual acuity is normal and the lesion remains undetected throughout the patient's life. In other cases, vision becomes impaired either from distortion of the macula or retinal detachment.

Signs

External   The eye is invariably white.

Slitlamp   The anterior chamber is quiet.

Vitreous A few cells may be seen in the retrovitral space.

Fundus The granuloma is white and hemispherical and is located at or anterior to the equator in any quadrant of the eye (*Figure 5.8*). The lesion is frequently associated with vitreous bands which extend to the posterior fundus. In severe cases a fold of retina joins the granuloma to the optic nerve head.

Clinical course and complications

In the majority of cases the visual prognosis is excellent. In some eyes with severe involvement, vision may become impaired due to the following tractional phenomena.

Heterotopia of the macula The traction bands connecting the granuloma with the optic nerve head may pull the blood vessels off the disc towards the lesion and also distort the macula. The 'dragging' of the macula may give rise to a pseudoexotropia.

Retinal detachment Both tractional and rhegmatogenous retinal detachments may develop as a result of contraction of vitreoretinal membranes and bands. Rhegmatogenous detachments are frequently caused by retinal dialyses.

Differential diagnosis

Retrolental fibroplasia (*Figure 5.9*) Both ocular toxocariasis and retrolental fibroplasia may cause 'dragging' of the disc and macula. However, in the former the 'dragging' can be in any direction because the granuloma does not have a predilection for the temporal retinal periphery as does retrolental fibroplasia. In addition, patients with retrolental fibroplasia invariably have bilateral lesions as well as a past history of prematurity and supplemental oxygen administration.

Congenital falciform retinal fold This classically begins at the optic disc and radiates to a large fibrous extension in the periphery. However, in contrast to the retinal fold in ocular toxocariasis, it is always associated with persistence of the hyaloid system.

Pars planitis An inferiorly located granuloma with a few cells in the retrolental space may, on cursory examination, be confused with pars planitis. However, the latter is usually bilateral and is associated with a more severe vitritis (*see* Chapter 8).

Management of ocular toxocariasis

Nil The majority of granulomas in quiet eyes require no specific therapy as the disease is 'burnt out'. Patients with dense vitreous membranes

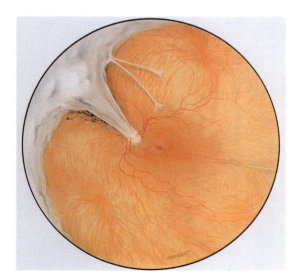

Figure 5.8 Peripheral toxocaral granuloma

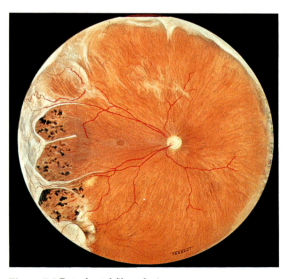

Figure 5.9 Retrolental fibroplasia

should, however, be observed in case they develop retinal detachment.

Medical   Anti-helminthic drugs such as thiabendazole and diethylcarbamazine are of minimal value in treating toxocaral endophthalmitis and they may even result in increased inflammation due to death of the toxocara organism. The majority of cases of endophthalmitis will respond well to a course of systemic or periocular steroids.

Scleral buckling surgery   Eyes with rhegmatogenous retinal detachments may respond to conventional scleral buckling procedures.

Pars plana vitrectomy   is indicated for the following reasons:

1 Endophthalmitis—eyes with chronic intraocular inflammation unresponsive to medical therapy may benefit from pars plana vitrectomy. Theoretically, the operation removes the larval antigen from the vitreous and makes the eye more quiet.
2 Retrolental cyclitic membrane—this can be excised with a vitreous cutter and the optical pathway restored. In addition vitrectomy may prevent the subsequent development of phthisis bulbi.
3 Vitreoretinal traction—vitrectomy may relieve vitreoretinal traction involving the macula, as well as correcting tractional retinal detachment.

Prophylaxis

Puppies should be dewormed with piperazine.

Diffuse unilateral subacute neuroretinitis

Introduction

Diffuse unilateral subacute neuroretinitis (DUSN) is thought to be caused by a common intestinal roundworm of lower carnivores, including raccoons and skunks, called *Baylisascaris procoynis*. This very rare disease affects mainly children and young adults.

Clinical features

Symptoms

The initial symptom is loss of central vision in one eye.

Signs

External   Nil.

Slitlamp   Nil.

Vitreous   A vitritis is frequently present.

Fundus   Multiple variably sized patches of grey-white outer retinal lesions occur in crops. In some cases they clear within several days without sequelae and in others they leave behind focal chorioretinal scars. In some eyes, a motile, non-segmented, tapered worm is observed moving under the retina. Swelling of the optic nerve head is also seen in about 20% of eyes.

Clinical course and complications

About 50% of eyes have a visual acuity of 6/60 or less due to narrowing of the retinal vessels, diffuse degeneration of the retinal pigment epithelium, and optic atrophy.

Management

In some cases the worm can be destroyed by photocoagulation.

Further reading

Toxoplasmosis
CHANDLER, S.H. (1979) Ocular abnormalities associated with intrauterine infections. *Perspectives in Ophthalmology*, **3**, 249–257
COTLIAR, A.M. and FRIEDMAN, A.H. (1982) Subretinal neovascularization in ocular toxoplasmosis. *British Journal of Ophthalmology*, **66**, 524–529
DOFT, B.H. and GASS, J.D.M. (1985) Punctate outer retinal toxoplasmosis. *Archives of Ophthalmology*, **103**, 1335–1336
DUTTON, G.N. and HAY, J. (1983) Toxoplasmic retinochoroiditis—current concepts in pathogenesis. *Transactions of the Ophthalmological Society of the United Kingdom*, **103**, 503–507

FITZGERALD, C.R. (1980) Pars plana vitrectomy for vitreous opacities secondary to presumed toxoplasmosis. *Archives of Ophthalmology*, **98**, 321–323

FOLK, J.C. and LOBES, L.A. (1984) Presumed toxoplasmic papillitis. *Ophthalmology*, **91**, 64–67

FRIEDMANN, C.T. and KNOX, D.L. (1969) Variations in recurrent active toxoplasmic retinochoroiditis. *Archives of Ophthalmology*, **81**, 481–493

GILES, C.L. (1971) Pyrimethamine (Daraprim) in the treatment of toxoplasmic uveitis. *Survey of Ophthalmology*, **16**, 88–91

MICHELSON, J.B., SHIELDS, J.A., FEDERMAN, J.L. *et al.* (1978) Retinitis secondary to acquired systemic toxoplasmosis with isolation of the parasite. *American Journal of Ophthalmology*, **86**, 548–552

NOZIK, R.A. (1977) Results of treatment of ocular toxoplasmosis with injectable corticosteroids. *Ophthalmology*, **83**, 811–818

O'CONNOR, G.R. and FRENKEL, J.K. (EDITORIAL) (1976) Dangers of steroid treatment in toxoplasmosis. *Archives of Ophthalmology*, **95**, 213

PERKINS, E.S. (1973) Ocular toxoplasmosis. *British Journal of Ophthalmology*, **57**, 1–17

SAARI, M., VOURRE, I., NIMINEN, H. *et al.* (1976) Acquired toxoplasmic chorioretinitis. *Archives of Ophthalmology*, **94**, 1485–1490

STERN, G.A. and ROMANO, P.E. (1978) Congenital toxoplasmosis. Possible occurrence in siblings. *Archives of Ophthalmology*, **96**, 615–618

TABBARA, K.F. and O'CONNOR, G.R. (1980) Treatment of ocular toxoplasmosis with clindamycin and sulfadiazine. *Ophthalmology*, **87**, 129–134

TATE, G.W. and MARTIN, R.G. (1977) Clindamycin in the treatment of human ocular toxoplasmosis. *Canadian Journal of Ophthalmology*, **12**, 188–191

Toxocariasis

BELMONT, J.B., IRVINE, A., BENSON, W. *et al.* (1982) Vitrectomy in ocular toxocariasis. *Archives of Ophthalmology*, **100**, 1912–1915

BIGLAN, A.W., GLICKMAN, L.T. and LOBES, L.A.JR (1979) Serum and vitreous toxocara antibody in nematode endophthalmitis. *American Journal of Ophthalmology*, **88**, 898–901

BYERS, B. and KIMURA, S. (1974) Uveitis after death of a larva in the vitreous cavity. *American Journal of Ophthalmology*, **77**, 63–66

DUGUID, I.M. (1961) Chronic endophthalmitis due to *Toxocara*. *British Journal of Ophthalmology*, **45**, 705–717

DUGUID, I.M. (1961) Features of ocular infestation by *Toxocara*. *British Journal of Ophthalmology*, **45**, 789–796

HAGLER, W.S., POLLARD, Z.F. and JARRETT, W.M. (1981) Results of surgery for *Toxocara canis*. *Ophthalmology*, **88**, 1081–1086

LUXEMBERG, M.N. (1979) An experimental approach to the study of intraocular *Toxocara canis*. *Transactions of the American Ophthalmological Society*, **77**, 542–602

POLLARD, Z.F., JARRETT, W.H., HAGLER, W.S. *et al.* (1979) ELISA for diagnosis of ocular toxocariasis. *Ophthalmology*, **86**, 743–749

SCHANTZ, P.M. and GLICKMAN, L.T. (1978) Toxocaral visceral larva migrans. *New England Journal of Medicine*, **298**, 436–439

WILKINSON, C.P. and WELCH, R.B. (1971) Intraocular toxocara. *American Journal of Ophthalmology*, **71**, 921–930

Diffuse unilateral subacute neuroretinitis

GASS, J.D.M. and BRAUNSTEIN, R.A. (1983) Further observations concerning the diffuse unilateral subacute neuroretinitis syndrome. *Archives of Ophthalmology*, **101**, 1689–1697

GASS, J.D.M., GILBERT, W.R., GUERRY, R.K. *et al.* (1978) Diffuse unilateral subacute neuroretinitis. *Ophthalmology*, **85**, 521–545

KAZAKOS, K.R., VESTRE, W.A. and KAZAKOS, E.A. (CORRESPONDENCE) (1984) Diffuse unilateral subacute neuroretinitis syndrome. *Archives of Ophthalmology*, **102**, 967–968

6

Viral infections

Herpes zoster uveitis

Introduction

Herpes zoster ophthalmicus (HZO) is an infection with the varicella-zoster virus of the first division of the trigeminal nerve. It accounts for between 10% and 25% of all dermatomal herpes zoster infections. The incidence of HZO increases with age and the infection is more common and usually more severe in immunosuppressed individuals and those with leukaemia and lymphoma. About 40% of patients with HZO develop an ipsilateral iridocyclitis usually within two weeks of the onset of the rash. Those with a vesicular eruption on the tip of the nose (*Figure 6.1*), from involvement of the external nasal branch of the nasociliary nerve (Hutchinson's sign), are at particular risk.

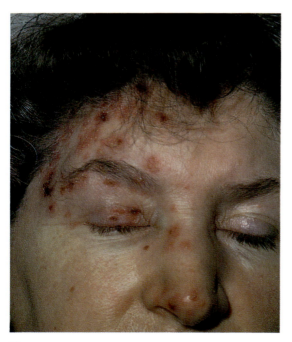

Figure 6.1 Hutchinson's sign

Clinical features

Symptoms

The symptoms are usually overshadowed by ocular pain caused by skin involvement, although occasionally severe ocular pain is due to a sudden rise in intraocular pressure.

Signs

External   The typical rash of HZO is present and the eye is usually injected due to associated conjunctivitis or episcleritis.

Slitlamp   The iridocyclitis is non-granulomatous with small keratic precipitates. The anterior chamber reaction is usually fairly mild with a faint flare and a moderate number of cells, although very occasionally severe iris ischaemia causes hypopyon which may be tinged with blood.

Note   Various forms of keratitis may also be present.

Vitreous   Cells are present in the anterior vitreous.

Fundus   This is usually normal, although a very small minority of cases show a retinitis characterized by yellow retinal exudates, retinal haemorrhages and vascular sheathing.

Clinical course and complications

Unless treated vigorously with topical steroids the anterior uveitis becomes chronic. The main complications of anterior uveitis are:

Iris atrophy (Figure 6.2)   About 20% of cases develop distortion of the pupil followed a few days later by iris atrophy, characterized by sectorial loss of the iris pigment epithelium which can be seen on transillumination. Fluorescein angiography of the iris shows occluded blood vessels at the site of atrophy.

Note   The iris atrophy from herpes simplex iritis is smaller, more sharply defined and has scalloped borders. Fluorescein angiography shows patent vessels in the involved area.

Secondary glaucoma   About 10% of eyes develop a rise in intraocular pressure which can sometimes be abrupt. The pressure elevation is caused by a combination of inflammation of the trabecular meshwork (trabeculitis) and trabecular obstruction by inflammatory debris.

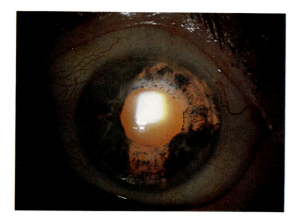

Figure 6.2 Iris atrophy due to herpes zoster

Secondary cataract   This develops in a few patients with chronic anterior uveitis.

Phthisis   This is very rare and is caused by severe ischaemia of the ciliary body.

Management

Steroids   In most cases treatment with topical steroids has to be continued for several months and then tapered very gradually. Systemic therapy is indicated in patients with posterior segment involvement.

Cycloplegics   These should be used together with steroids to prevent the formation of posterior synechiae.

Antivirals   Antivirals in the form of oral acyclovir 600 mg five times a day for 10 days may reduce both the incidence as well as the duration of anterior uveitis.

Differential diagnosis

Although, in the majority of cases the diagnosis is straightforward, it is important to remember that severe uveitis may occur in patients with only a slight rash anywhere on the forehead. In these cases, the initial diagnosis of HZO might have been missed and the patient may present several months later with a chronic unilateral iridocyclitis. In order not to miss the diagnosis, always think of the possibility of HZO as a cause of anterior uveitis and perform the following tests:

1 Test corneal sensation as this is frequently diminished following zoster keratitis.
2 Examine the cornea for evidence of nummular lesions which may persist for many months.
3 Transilluminate the iris for evidence of atrophy.
4 Examine the patient's scalp at the hairline for evidence of post-herpetic scarring and pigmentation.

Herpes simplex anterior uveitis

Introduction

Controversy exists concerning the occurrence of herpes simplex uveitis in the absence of keratitis.

Some authorities believe that this never occurs, whilst others are of the opinion that some cases of iridocyclitis are due to direct invasion of the anterior uvea by virus particles. In most eyes with herpes simplex keratitis and anterior uveitis, the latter is probably due to a hypersensitivity phenomenon, not associated with the presence of virus particles in the uvea.

Clinical features

Herpes simplex anterior uveitis occurs in three different settings.

Associated with dendritic or geographic ulceration

Signs

External   The eye is photophobic and slightly injected.

Slitlamp   An active fluorescein-staining corneal lesion is present (*Figure 6.3*). The associated anterior uveitis is acute and follows the development of keratitis by one or two days. Secondary glaucoma may occur in severe cases and recurrent attacks may cause iris atrophy.

> *Note*   The iris atrophy consists of small, sharply defined, areas with scalloped borders, in contrast to the larger segmental iris atrophy of herpes zoster.

Management

The keratitis is treated with topical antiviral agents. The pupil should be kept mobile to prevent posterior synechiae, but topical steroids should never be used in the presence of active epithelial keratitis.

Associated with disciform keratitis

Signs

External   The eye is usually white.

Slitlamp   A typical disciform keratitis consists of a central zone of epithelial oedema overlying an area of stromal thickening. Some eyes also show folds in Descemet's membrane. The anterior uveitis is usually mild with +1 or +2 aqueous cells. The keratic precipitates are small or medium in size and they are characteristically located on the back of the disciform lesion (*Figure 6.4*). Occasionally the intraocular pressure is elevated despite the presence of only mild uveitis.

Management

Treatment is with mydriatics and topical steroids.

Unassociated with keratitis

Signs

External   Nil apart from diminished corneal sensation in some patients. In these cases it seemed likely that the patient originally had a

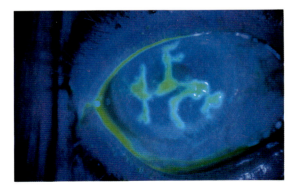

Figure 6.3 Large dendritic ulcer stained with fluorescein

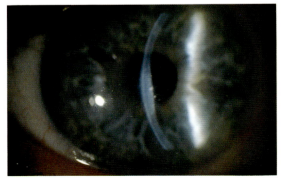

Figure 6.4 Disciform keratitis

corneal lesion, but all traces of the infection had disappeared by the time the diagnosis of uveitis was made and the only possible clue to previous keratitis was diminished corneal sensation. It is also possible that the uveitis is unassociated with a previous attack of keratitis.

Slitlamp   A mild to moderate anterior uveitis is present.

Management

Treatment is with topical steroids and mydriatics. The patient should be examined at frequent intervals to ensure that he does not develop a dendritic ulcer.

Herpes simplex retinitis

Introduction

Posterior segment involvement by the herpes simplex virus (HSV) is extremely rare. It may be congenital or acquired.

Congenital

This occurs in neonates with immature immunological systems. The infant becomes infected with HSV type 2 on passage through the birth canal and the retinitis is usually associated with generalized infection and encephalitis.

Acquired

This affects adults in two different clinical settings.

With encephalitis   Very rarely, retinitis occurs during the course of encephalitis caused by HSV type 1 in previously healthy individuals. The encephalitis, which may be fatal, presents with fever, headache, neck stiffness, and focal neurological signs. Retinitis usually presents early during the course of the disease.

With immunosuppression   Patients on chemotherapy for advanced malignancies, graft recipients maintained on immunosuppressive agents and patients with AIDS are at increased risk of HSV retinitis.

Clinical features

Both eyes are usually involved.

Signs

External   The eye is usually white.

Slitlamp   A mild anterior uveitis is common.

Vitreous   A vitritis is invariably present.

Fundus   The spectrum of fundus lesions includes: venous engorgement, flame-shaped haemorrhages, papillitis, retinal oedema, perivasculitis with vascular occlusion, and a hazy yellow-white necrotic retina.

Clinical course and complications

HSV retinitis may have a devastating effect on vision due to the development of either exudative or rhegmatogenous retinal detachment. If the retinitis heals, granular hyperpigmentation develops.

Management

Treatment is with: intravenous acyclovir 5–7.5 mg/kg eight-hourly for 1 week or intravenous vidarabine 15 mg/kg per day for 10 days.

Differential diagnosis

Cytomegalovirus retinitis   Both cytomegalovirus (CMV) and HSV retinitis occur in immunocompromised patients and the clinical appearance may be similar, particularly during the late stages, although there is usually less haemorrhage in HSV retinitis. In some cases the differentiation can only be made on the basis of associated non-ocular clinical findings, viral cultures, and serological tests.

Acute retinal necrosis (ARN)   Patients with ARN are normal immunologically and retinal haemorrhage is not as common as in HSV retinitis (*see* Chapter 9).

> *Note*   It now seems likely that some cases of ARN are in fact caused by a herpes virus.

Acquired cytomegalovirus infections

Systemic predispositions

Cytomegalovirus (CMV) retinitis is a rare chronic diffuse exudative infection of the retina caused by the CMV virus which occurs, with rare exceptions, in patients with an impaired immune system due to one of the following causes:

AIDS—see later.
Cytotoxic chemotherapy—for malignancies, such as leukaemia and lymphoma.
Long-term immunosuppression—following organ transplantation.

Ocular features

Symptoms

Blurred vision if the posterior pole is involved.

Signs

External   The eye is white.

Anterior chamber   Mild anterior uveitis is common.

Vitreous   A mild vitritis is common but never severe.

Fundus   The earliest findings are white lesions (*Figure 6.5a*), similar to cotton-wool spots. These are followed by the appearance of geographical, yellow-white granular areas which represent areas of full-thickness retinal necrosis and oedema (*Figure 6.5b*) which starts either peripherally (*Figure 6.6*) or at the posterior pole. Later the

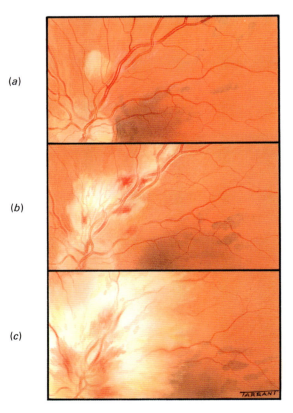

(a)

(b)

(c)

Figure 6.5 Progression of CMV retinitis

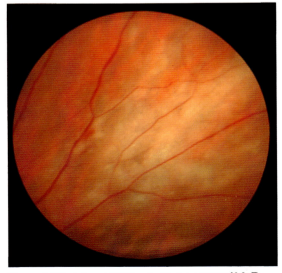

Figure 6.6 Peripheral CMV retinitis (courtesy of Mr D. Spalton)

lesions coalesce (*Figure 6.5c*) and are associated with retinal haemorrhages and vasculitis at their advancing border. The associated retinal nerve fibre haemorrhages may resemble retinal branch vein occlusions. The infective process spreads slowly and relentlessly along the course of the retinal blood vessels to involve the entire fundus (*Figure 6.7*) and leads to total retinal atrophy and, occasionally, also involvement of the optic nerve. Some eyes develop exudative or rhegmatogenous retinal detachments.

Management

A recent study has shown that treatment with intravenous dihydroxypropoxymethyl guanine causes regression in some cases.

Differential diagnosis

Acute retinal necrosis This usually affects healthy patients. It spreads more quickly than CMV retinitis and is associated with less haemorrhage (*see* Chapter 9).

HSV retinitis Although HSV retinitis may occasionally occur in immunocompromised patients, it is more frequently associated with herpetic encephalitis. The retinal lesions may be very similar, particularly during the later stages, although the amount of haemorrhage is usually less in HSV retinitis.

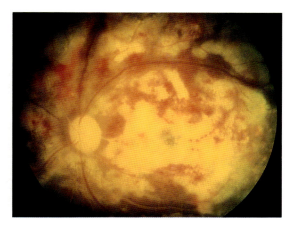

Figure 6.7 Extensive CMV retinitis (courtesy of Mr R. Marsh)

Congenital cytomegalovirus infection

Systemic features

Congenital CMV infection is acquired transplacentally and typically affects premature infants. The severely affected neonate may suffer from a whole range of abnormalities including low birth weight, hepatosplenomegaly, jaundice, purpura, thrombocytopenia, microcephaly, and pneumonitis. Involvement of the central nervous system may cause cerebral periventricular calcification, deafness, psychomotor retardation, and seizures.

Ocular features

Signs

External Anophthalmos, microphthalmos and cataract may be present.

Fundus Retinochoroiditis resembling toxoplasmosis is the most common finding. It is, however, usually multifocal and peripheral in location. Other findings include optic atrophy, optic nerve hypoplasia, and optic nerve coloboma.

Acquired immune deficiency syndrome

Systemic features

The acquired immune deficiency syndrome (AIDS) is defined by the occurrence of Kaposi's sarcoma or opportunistic infections, or both, in previously healthy persons less than 60 years of age whose immunosuppression has no known cause. The syndrome most commonly affects homosexual men, but it may also affect haemophiliacs, and Haitian immigrants to the United States. Female sexual partners of men with AIDS and infants of women in known risk groups from AIDS are also at risk. The virus HTLV-3 is the causative pathogen of this invariably fatal disease. The opportunistic infections in AIDS include the following.

Protozoa

Pneumocystis carnii pneumonia.
Disseminated toxoplasmosis.

Viruses

Disseminated CMV.
Persistent invasive HSV.
Herpes zoster.
Epstein–Barr virus.
Adenovirus.

Fungi

Systemic cryptococcosis.
Oral and oesophageal candidiasis.

Bacteria

Mycobacterium avium-intracellulare.

Ocular features

Ocular complications occur in about 75% of AIDS patients.

Signs

External

Kaposi's sarcoma may involve the eyelids and conjunctiva. It appears as a bright red mass, most frequently in the lower fornix. Skin tumours appear as elevated, non-tender purple nodules.

Severe herpes zoster ophthalmicus can sometimes be an early manifestation of the disease.

Slitlamp The uveitis due to herpes zoster is usually severe and prolonged in AIDS patients.

Vitreous A vitritis is present in eyes with CMV retinitis, candida endophthalmitis, and toxoplasmic retinitis.

Fundus

Cotton-wool spots identical to those seen in hypertension and diabetes are seen in about 50% of patients. They are usually transient and resolve over a period of four to six weeks. Some patients also develop scattered retinal nerve fibre haemorrhages, usually in the absence of cotton-wool spots. At present the cause of the cotton-wool spots and haemorrhages is unknown.

CMV retinitis (Figures 6.5, 6.6, 6.7) occurs in about 30% of homosexual AIDS patients and is the major cause of visual loss. Its appearance is a grave prognostic sign as most patients are dead within six to eight weeks.

> *Note* Much less common forms of retinitis in AIDS patients are caused by toxoplasmosis, candidiasis, HSV, and *Mycobacterium avium-intracellulare.*

Management

A temporary regression of CMV retinitis has been reported in some patients following intravenous administration of dihydroxypropoxymethyl guanine. Kaposi's sarcoma is sensitive to radiotherapy.

Rubella (German measles)

Systemic features

Serological studies have shown that about 15% of all women of childbearing age are susceptible to rubella. Transmission of the virus appears to require close contact and probably occurs through the respiratory route. Immunity following natural infection is longstanding. Fetal infection is probably the direct result of maternal viraemia (which may be clinical or subclinical) with seeding of the virus in the placenta. The risk to the fetus is closely related to the stage of gestation at the time of maternal infection. Fetal infection is about 50% during the first 8 weeks, 33% between the ninth and twelfth weeks, and about 10% between the thirteenth and twenty-fourth week. Each of the various organs that may be affected has its own period of susceptibility to the infection, after which no gross malformations are produced. Systemic complications of maternal rubella include: spontaneous abortions, stillbirth, congenital heart malformations, deafness, microcephaly, mental retardation, hypotonia, hepatosplenomegaly, thrombocytopenic purpura, and pneumonitis.

Ocular features

Signs

External   Anterior segment complications include cataract, microphthalmos, glaucoma, corneal haze, nystagmus, and strabismus.

Slitlamp   At the time of cataract extraction, the virus may be released from the lens into the aqueous humour and cause a severe anterior uveitis. The intraocular inflammation may be prolonged and give rise to a cyclitic membrane, which in turn may cause detachment of the ciliary body and phthisis bulbi.

Fundus   A diffuse chorioretinopathy which is probably due to viral involvement of the cells of the retinal pigment epithelium is a common finding. The retina has a 'salt-and-pepper' appearance, consisting of discrete, patchy, areas of hyperpigmentation interspersed with similar patches of depigmentation (*Figure 6.8*). The

inflammation is usually inactive when the chorioretinopathy is first detected. Visual acuity is generally not affected, although choroidal neovascularization may develop in a very small number of cases. A few cases may also show optic atrophy.

Rubeola (measles)

Systemic features

Subacute sclerosing panencephalitis is a lethal neurological disorder which typically affects children and young adults several months or even years following apparent recovery from measles. It usually starts with personality or behavioural changes, followed by dementia, seizures, myoclonus, muscle weakness, and eventually death within two years.

Ocular features

Signs

External   Nil.

Slitlamp   Nil.

Fundus   The typical lesion which occurs in about 50% of patients consists of a focal macular or paramacular retinitis manifest as a 'ground-glass' whitening of the retina. Other features include optic atrophy and papilloedema.

Management

There is no effective treatment.

Other viruses

Infectious mononucleosis

Glandular fever is occasionally associated with a mild bilateral transient anterior uveitis and rarely a chorioretinitis.

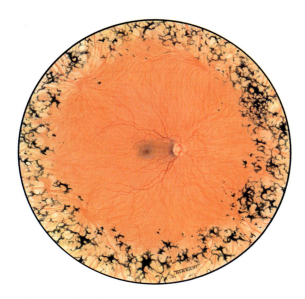

Figure 6.8 Rubella chorioretinopathy

Influenza

Both influenza and parainfluenza viruses may cause a transient mild bilateral anterior uveitis which usually develops about two weeks after an attack of influenza.

References

Herpes zoster uveitis

COBO, L.M., FOULKS, G.N., LIESEGANG, T. *et al.* (1985) Oral acyclovir in the therapy of acute herpes zoster ophthalmicus. *Ophthalmology*, **92**, 1574–1582

COLES, E.L., MEISLER, D.M., CALABRESE, L.H. *et al.* (1984) Herpes zoster ophthalmicus and acquired immune deficiency syndrome. *Archives of Ophthalmology*, **102**, 1027–1029

HEDGES, T.R. and ALBERT, D.M. (1982) The progression of the ocular abnormalities of herpes zoster: Histopathologic observations of nine cases. *Ophthalmology*, **89**, 165–176

LIESEGANG, T.J. (1985) Corneal complications from herpes zoster ophthalmicus. *Ophthalmology*, **92**, 316–324

LIGHTMAN, S., MARSH, R.J. and POWELL, D. (1981) Herpes zoster ophthalmicus: a medical review. *British Journal of Ophthalmology*, **65**, 539–541

McGILL, J., CHAPMAN, C. and MAHAKASINGHAM, M. (1983) Acyclovir therapy in herpes zoster infection—a practical guide. *Transactions of the Ophthalmological Society of the United Kingdom*, **103**, 111–114

MARSH, R.J. (1976) Current management of herpes zoster ophthalmicus. *Archives of Ophthalmology*, **96**, 334–337

WOMACK, L.W. and LIESEGANG, T.J. (1983) Complications of herpes zoster ophthalmicus. *Archives of Ophthalmology*, **101**, 42–45

Herpes simplex anterior uveitis

MARTENET, A.C. (1981) Role of viruses in uveitis. *Transactions of the Ophthalmological Society of the United Kingdom*, **101**, 308–311

OH, J.O. (1976) Primary and secondary herpes simplex uveitis in rabbits. *Survey of Ophthalmology*, **21**, 178–184

Herpes simplex retinitis

GRUTZMACHER, R.D., HENDERSON, D., MCDONALD, P.J. *et al.* (1983) Herpes simplex chorioretinitis in a healthy adult. *American Journal of Ophthalmology*, **96**, 788–796

PARTAMIAN, L.G., MORSE, P.H. and KLEIN, H.Z. (1981) Herpes simplex type 1 retinitis in an adult with systemic herpes zoster. *American Journal of Ophthalmology*, **92**, 215–220

PEPOSE, J.S., KREIGER, A.E., TOMIYASU, U. *et al.* (1985) Immunocytologic localization of herpes simplex type 1

viral antigens in herpetic retinitis and encephalitis in an adult. *Ophthalmology*, **92**, 160–166

UNINSKY, E., JAMPOL, L.M., KAUFMAN, S. *et al.* (1983) Disseminated herpes simplex infection with retinitis in a renal allograft recipient. *Ophthalmology*, **90**, 175–178

Cytomegalovirus infection

BERGER, B.B., WEINBERG, R.S. and TESSLER, H. (1979) Bilateral cytomegalovirus panuveitis after high dose corticosteroid therapy. *American Journal of Ophthalmology*, **88**, 1020–1025

DEVENECIA, G., ZU RHEIM, G.M., PRATT, M.V. *et al.* (1971) Cytomegalic inclusion retinitis in an adult. *Archives of Ophthalmology*, **86**, 44–57

MEREDITH, T.A., AABERG, T.M. and REESER, F.H. (1979) Rhegmatogenous retinal detachment complicating cytomegalovirus retinitis. *American Journal of Ophthalmology*, **87**, 793–796

PALESTINE, A.G., STEVENS, G., LANE, H.C. *et al.* (1986) Treatment of cytomegalovirus retinitis with dihydroxypropoxymethyl guanine. *American Journal of Ophthalmology*, **101**, 95–101

Acquired immune deficiency syndrome

BACHMAN, D.M., RODRIGUES, M.M. and CHU, F. (1982) Culture proven cytomegalovirus retinitis in a homosexual man with the acquired immune deficiency syndrome. *Ophthalmology*, **89**, 797–804

FREEMAN, W.R., LERNER, C.W., MINES, J.A. *et al.* (1984) A prospective study of the ophthalmic findings in the acquired immune deficiency syndrome. *American Journal of Ophthalmology*, **97**, 133–142

HOLLAND, G.N., GOTTLIEB, M.S., YEE, R.D. *et al.* (1982) Ocular disorders associated with a new severe acquired cellular immunodeficiency syndrome. *American Journal of Ophthalmology*, **93**, 393–402

HOLLAND, G.N., PEPOSE, J.S., PETTIT, T.H. *et al.* (1983) Acquired immune deficiency syndrome. Ocular manifestations. *Ophthalmology*, **90**, 859–873

KHADEM, M., KALISH, S.B., GOLDSMITH, J. *et al.* (1984) Ophthalmic findings in acquired immune deficiency syndrome (AIDS). *Archives of Ophthalmology*, **102**, 201–206

NEWMAN, N.M., MANDEL, M.R., GULLETT, J. *et al.* (1983) Clinical and histologic findings in opportunistic ocular infections. Part of a new syndrome of acquired immunodeficiency. *Archives of Ophthalmology*, **101**, 396–401

PALESTINE, A.G., RODRIGUEZ, M.M., MACHER, A.M. *et al.* (1984) Ophthalmic involvement in acquired immune deficiency syndrome. *Ophthalmology*, **91**, 1092–1099

ROSENBERG, P.R., ULISS, A.E., FRIEDLAND, G.H. *et al.* (1983) Acquired immunodeficiency syndrome. Ophthalmic manifestations in ambulatory patients. *Ophthalmology*, **90**, 874–878

7

Fungal infections

Presumed ocular histoplasmosis syndrome

Introduction

Histoplasmosis is a fungal infection caused by *Histoplasma capsulatum*. The disease is acquired by inhalation and the organisms pass via the blood stream to the spleen, liver and, on occasion, to the choroid, setting up multiple foci of granulomatous inflammation. In the vast majority of patients, the fungaemia is innocuous and asymptomatic as the organisms disappear after a few weeks. A small minority of patients with severe disseminated systemic histoplasmosis develop an endophthalmitis.

Although the presumed ocular histoplasmosis syndrome (POHS) has never been reported in patients with active disseminated systemic histoplasmosis, the disease has an increased prevalence in areas where histoplasmosis is endemic, such as the Mississippi–Ohio–Missouri river valley. So far *Histoplasma capsulatum* has not been recovered from an eye with POHS.

> *Note* A syndrome identical to POHS has been reported in the United Kingdom where histoplasmosis does not occur.

Diagnostic tests

Histoplasma skin test This is positive in about 90% of patients with POHS.

Complement fixation test These are of limited value because they usually become negative several years after the original infection.

X-rays In some patients, plain X-rays will show old calcified granulomas in the lungs and spleen.

Tissue typing Patients with POHS, particularly if associated with maculopathy, have an increased prevalence of HLA-B7.

Fundus fluorescein angiography This is extremely useful in detecting early subretinal neovascular membranes.

Clinical features

Symptoms

The POHS is asymptomatic unless it causes a maculopathy. The earliest symptom of macular involvement is metamorphopsia.

Signs

Both eyes are usually affected.

External Nil.

Slitlamp Normal.

Vitreous Uninvolved.

Fundus Four types of lesion are observed (*Figure 7.1*).

Atrophic spots called 'histo spots' consist of roundish, slightly irregular, yellowish-white lesions measuring between 0.2 and 0.7 disc diameters in size. Small pigment clumps may be

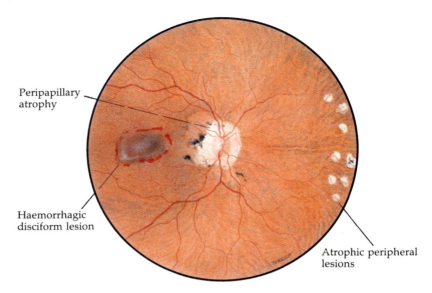

Peripapillary atrophy

Haemorrhagic disciform lesion

Atrophic peripheral lesions

Figure 7.1 Presumed ocular histoplasmosis syndrome

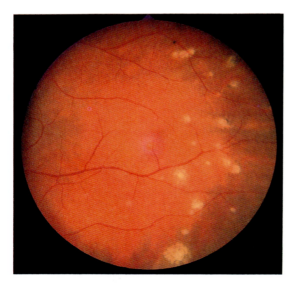

Figure 7.2 Peripheral 'histo spots' in presumed ocular histoplasmosis syndrome

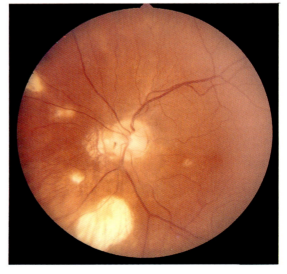

Figure 7.3 Peripapillary atrophy in presumed ocular histoplasmosis syndrome

present within or at the margins of the scars although some spots are not associated with pigmentation (*Figure 7.2*). The lesions are scattered in the mid-retinal periphery and the posterior pole.

> *Note* 'Histo spots' are probably caused by subclinical histoplasmosis during childhood when the fungus caused a multifocal choroiditis which healed spontaneously leaving small areas of chorioretinal atrophy.

Peripapillary atrophy (Figure 7.3) is characterized, most frequently, by a diffuse circumferential choroidal atrophy extending up to 0.5 disc diameters beyond the border of the optic disc. Less commonly, the peripapillary lesions are irregular and punched out, resembling the peripheral spots. In some eyes both diffuse and focal lesions are seen.

Linear streaks of chorioretinal atrophy in the fundus periphery have recently been described.

Subretinal choroidal neovascularization is a late manifestation of POHS which usually develops between the ages of 20 and 45 years. In the majority of cases, the neovascular membranes are associated with an old macular 'histo spot', although occasionally they develop within a peripapillary lesion. Very rarely the membranes occur in the absence of a pre-existing scar and they have also been reported in association with peripheral 'histo spots'.

> *Note* Histological studies have confirmed that the neovascular membranes are associated with breaks in Bruch's membrane which allow the ingrowth of neovascular tissue from the choriocapillaris into the subpigment epithelial space.

Clinical course and complications

The clinical course of maculopathy is variable.

Serous detachment The neovascular membrane may initially leak fluid and give rise to metamorphopsia, blurring of central vision and a positive relative scotoma. Careful slitlamp biomicroscopy with a fundus contact lens shows that the macula is elevated by serous fluid and an underlying focal yellow-white or grey lesion. In some eyes the subretinal fluid absorbs spontaneously and visual symptoms regress.

Haemorrhagic detachment Frequently, a dark green-black ring develops on the surface of the yellow-white lesion and bleeding occurs into the subsensory retinal space (*Figure 7.4*) causing a marked drop in visual acuity. In a few eyes, the subretinal haemorrhage resolves and visual acuity improves.

Disciform scar In some eyes, the initial neovascular complex remains active for about 2 years giving rise to repeated haemorrhages. This finally causes a profound and permanent impairment of central vision due to the development of a fibrous disciform scar at the fovea.

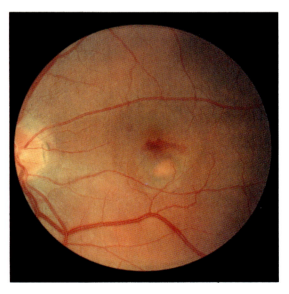

Figure 7.4 Subretinal neovascularization in presumed ocular histoplasmosis syndrome (courtesy of Dr P. Morse)

Note Patients with maculopathy in one eye and an asymptomatic atrophic macular scar in the other eye are likely to develop a disciform lesion in the second eye. They should therefore test themselves every day with an Amsler grid to detect early metamorphopsia.

Management

The mainstay of treatment of subretinal neovascular membranes in eyes with POHS is argon laser photocoagulation. Without treatment, 60% of eyes have a final visual acuity of less than 6/60. Most favourable results of photocoagulation are in eyes with neovascular complexes not closer than 0.25 disc diameter from the centre of the fovea and with intact capillary free zones. Pre-treatment fundus fluorescein angiography is vital in evaluating the extent and location of neovascular membranes.

Differential diagnosis

Contrary to all other types of posterior uveitis, eyes with POHS have a clear vitreous. Some other non-inflammatory disorders that might be considered in the differential diagnosis include the following:

Myopic degeneration The atrophic spots in myopia are usually whiter, more punched out and located only at the posterior pole.

Angioid streaks The 'salmon spots' in eyes with angioid streaks may be similar to 'histo spots'. However, patients with angioid streaks frequently have an associated systemic disorder such as pseudoxanthoma elasticum.

Candidiasis

Systemic predispositions

Candida albicans, a yeast-like fungus, is a frequent commensal of the human skin, mouth, gastrointestinal tract, and vagina. Candidiasis is an opportunistic infection in which the organism acquires pathogenic properties. Candidaemia, which may result in ocular involvement, occurs in three main groups of patients:

1 Drug addicts may acquire the disease through the use of non-sterile needles and syringes. Not infrequently they have no obvious evidence of disseminated candidiasis and negative blood and urine cultures for *Candida*. In this group of patients the diagnosis may be missed unless the skin is carefully examined for evidence of injection site scars.
2 Patients with long-term indwelling catheters used for haemodialysis or intravenous nutrition following extensive bowel surgery are at increased risk.
3 'Compromised host'—these are usually severely debilitated patients with decreased immunity either from an underlying systemic disease (AIDS, malignancies) and/or patients on long-term treatment with drugs such as antibiotics, steroids, and cytotoxic agents.

Ocular features

Symptoms

Depending on the location of the initial lesion, the symptoms include pain, photophobia, floaters, and blurred vision. Both eyes are usually involved but the severity of infection is frequently asymmetrical.

Signs

External The eye is usually white although occasionally a scleritis is present.

Slitlamp Anterior uveitis is common and may be associated with a hypopyon.

Note In patients with severe anterior uveitis, the possibility of an underlying chorioretinitis may be overlooked.

Fundus Although the initial foci involve the choroid, the organisms soon invade the retina and gives rise to a multifocal retinitis manifest as small, round, white, slightly elevated lesions with indistinct borders (*Figure 7.5a*). As the lesions grow they may be associated with haemorrhages which, on occasion, have pale centres (Roth's spots). With appropriate antifungal therapy, the retinal lesions heal leaving behind a faint glial scar or a focal defect in the retinal pigment epithelium.

Vitreous Unless antifungal therapy is instituted, the small retinal lesions enlarge and extend into the vitreous gel giving rise to floating white 'puff-ball' or 'cotton-ball' colonies (*Figure 7.5b*). Several colonies joined together by opalescent strands are referred to as a 'string of pearls' (*Figure 7.5c*).

Clinical course and complications

Some mild cases of retinitis (*Figure 7.6*) heal spontaneously. Advanced cases are characterized by a vitreoretinal abscess and severe retinal necrosis (*Figure 7.7*). Secondary vitreous organization may give rise to a tractional retinal detachment.

Medical treatment

In the past, amphotericin B was the mainstay of therapy for ocular candidiasis. However, newer

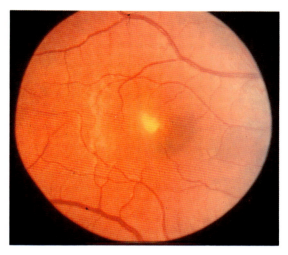

Figure 7.6 Mild focal candida retinitis (courtesy of Mr R. Marsh)

(a)

(b)

(c)

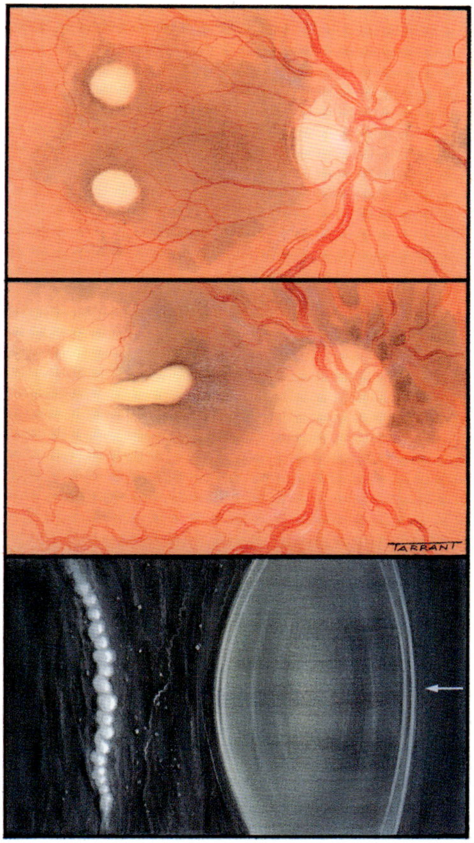

Figure 7.5 Progression of ocular candidiasis: (*a*) multifocal retinitis; (*b*) extension into vitreous; (*c*) 'string of pearls'

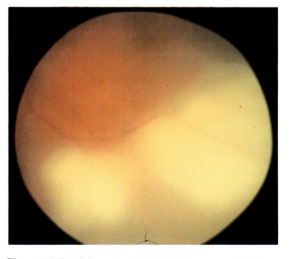

Figure 7.7 Candida endophthalmitis (courtesy of Mr R. Marsh)

and less toxic drugs are now available which can be given orally. Initial treatment should be with a combination of 5-fluorocytosine (flucytosine) 150 mg/kg per day and ketoconazole 200 mg/kg per day for three weeks. Alternative therapy in resistant cases is intravenous amphotericin B in 5% dextrose given over a period of several days until a cumulative dose of 200 mg has been reached. The initial dose is 5 mg/day and after a few days this can be increased to 20 mg/day.

Note
1 Steroids should not be used as they will make the infection worse.
2 Most cases with severe vitreous involvement do badly due to a combination of late diagnosis and poor penetration of antifungal drugs into the vitreous gel.

Pars plana vitrectomy

Cases with moderate to severe vitreous involvement (endophthalmitis) are best treated by pars plana vitrectomy and injection of 5 µg of amphotericin B into the central vitreous cavity. At the time of vitrectomy, smears and cultures should be taken to confirm the diagnosis and test the sensitivity of the organisms to antifungal agents.

Differential diagnosis

Cotton-wool spots   The small foci of early retinitis are rounder than cotton-wool spots and are associated with an overlying vitreous haze.

Pars planitis   The vitreous 'puff-balls' may resemble the 'snowballs' of pars planitis (*see Figure 1.14*). However, snowbanking is absent in candidiasis.

Toxoplasmosis   Candida retinitis is not associated with a healed chorioretinal scar. Toxoplasmic retinochoroiditis remains confined to the retina whereas the lesions caused by *Candida* first bulge into and then float in the vitreous cavity.

CMV retinitis   Although both candidiasis and CMV retinitis may affect immunocompromised patients, the latter is more diffuse and is associated with haemorrhages and only a mild vitritis (*see* Chapter 6).

Further reading

Histoplasmosis

ARCHER, D.B., MAGUIRE, C.J.F. and NEWELL, F.W. (1975) Multifocal choroiditis. *Transactions of the Ophthalmological Society of the United Kingdom*, **95**, 184–191

DREYER, R.F. and GASS, J.D.M. (1984) Multifocal choroiditis and panuveitis. *Archives of Ophthalmology*, **102**, 1776–1784

GANLEY, J.P. (1984) Epidemiology of presumed ocular histoplasmosis. *Archives of Ophthalmology*, **102**, 1754–1756

KAHILL, M.K. (1982) Histopathology of presumed ocular histoplasmosis. *American Journal of Ophthalmology*, **94**, 369–376

KLEIN, M.L. and FINE, S.L. (1977) Natural history of choroidal neovascular membranes in ocular histoplasmosis. *Perspectives in Ophthalmology*, **1**, 137–139

LEWIS, M.L., VANNEWKIRK, M.R. and GASS, J.D.M. (1980) Follow-up study of presumed ocular histoplasmosis syndrome. *Ophthalmology*, **87**, 390–398

MACHER, A., RODRIGUES, M.M., KAPLAN, W. et al. (1985) Disseminated bilateral choroiditis due to *Histoplasma capsulatum* in a patient with acquired immune deficiency syndrome. *Ophthalmology*, **92**, 1159–1164

MEREDITH, T.A., GREEN, W.R., KEY, S.N. et al. (1977) Ocular histoplasmosis: Clinicopathological correlation in three cases. *Survey of Ophthalmology*, **22**, 189–205

ROTH, A.M. (1977) Histoplasma capsulatum in the presumed ocular histoplasmosis syndrome. *American Journal of Ophthalmology*, **84**, 293–298

SCHLAEGEL, T.F.JR (1977) The prognosis in the presumed ocular histoplasmosis syndrome. *Perspectives in Ophthalmology*, **1**, 140–145

SCHLAEGEL, T.F.JR (1977) The principles of partial photocoagulation of the presumed ocular histoplasmosis syndrome. *Perspectives in Ophthalmology*, **1**, 119–124

SMITH, R.E. (1977) Ocular histoplasmosis—signs and symptoms. *Perspectives in Ophthalmology*, **1**, 101–106

SMITH, R.E. (1977) Differential diagnosis of ocular histoplasmosis. *Perspectives in Ophthalmology*, **1**, 107–110

SMITH, R.E. (1981) Studies in the presumed ocular histoplasmosis syndrome. *Transactions of the Ophthalmological Society of the United Kingdom*, **101**, 328–334

WATZKE, R.C. and CLAUSSEN, R.W. (1981) The long-term course of multifocal choroiditis (presumed ocular histoplasmosis). *American Journal of Ophthalmology*, **91**, 750–760

Candidiasis

AGUILAR, G.L., BLUMENKRANZ, M.S., EGBERT, P.R. et al. (1979) Candida endophthalmitis after intravenous drug abuse. *Archives of Ophthalmology*, **97**, 96–102

BROWNSTEIN, S., MAHONEY-KINSNER, J. and HARRIS, R. (1983) Ocular candida with pale centre haemorrhages. *Archives of Ophthalmology*, **101**, 1745–1748

McDONNELL, P.J., McDONNELL, J.M., BROWN, R.H. *et al.* (1985) Ocular involvement in patients with fungal infections. *Ophthalmology*, **92**, 706–709

PARKE, D.W. III, JONES, D.B. and GENTRY, L.O. (1982) Endogenous endophthalmitis among patients with candidemia. *Ophthalmology*, **89**, 789–796

SALMON, J.F., PARTRIDGE, B.M. and SPALTON, D.J. (1983) Candida endophthalmitis in a heroin addict. *British Journal of Ophthalmology*, **67**, 306–309

SERVANT, J.B., DUTTON, G.N., ONG-TONE, L. *et al.* (1985) Candida endophthalmitis in Glaswegian heroin addicts: Reports of an epidemic. *Transactions of the Ophthalmological Society of the United Kingdom*, **104**, 297–308

8

Common idiopathic specific uveitis entities

Fuchs' uveitis syndrome

Introduction

Fuchs' uveitis syndrome (FUS) or Fuchs' heterochromic cyclitis is a chronic non-granulomatous anterior uveitis which has an insidious onset. It typically affects one eye of a middle-aged adult, although it can also occur during childhood and may very occasionally be bilateral. Although FUS accounts for about 2% of all cases of uveitis, it is probably misdiagnosed and overtreated more than any other uveitis entity. The heterochromia (difference in iris colour) may be absent in some patients or it may be difficult to detect, particularly in brown-eyed individuals, unless the patient is examined in daylight with undilated pupils.

Clinical features

Symptoms

The vast majority of patients are asymptomatic until the development of secondary cataract. A few patients complain of vitreous floaters and some notice a colour difference between the two eyes. Not infrequently the condition is detected by chance.

Signs

External   The eye is invariably white.

Slitlamp

Cornea   The keratic precipitates are characteristic and possibly pathognomonic. They are small,

round or stellate, grey-white in colour and are scattered throughout the corneal endothelium (*Figure 8.1* and *see Figure 1.3*). They may come and go but they never become confluent or pigmented. Feathery fibrin filaments may be seen interdisposed between the keratic precipitates.

Aqueous humour   A faint flare and cells (never more than +2) are usually present.

Iris
1 Posterior synechiae are invariably *absent*.

> *Note*   The presence of posterior synechiae excludes a diagnosis of FUS.

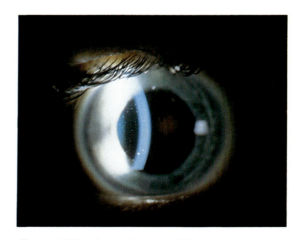

Figure 8.1 Keratic precipitates in FUS

2 Atrophy (*Figure 8.2*)—the typical findings are diffuse stromal atrophy which may be associated with patchy atrophy of the posterior pigment layer of the iris. In early cases the only abnormal finding is a loss of iris crypts. More advanced stromal atrophy makes the affected iris appear dull with loss of detail giving rise to a 'washed out' appearance, particularly in the pupillary zone. The patchy atrophy of the posterior pigment layer can be detected on iris transillumination (*see Figure 1.10*) and gaps in pigmented pupillary frill make the border of the pupil appear moth-eaten. The normal radial iris blood vessels appear prominent due to lack of stromal support.

3 Heterochromia—most frequently the affected eye is hypochromic although this is an inconsistent feature. In some patients it may be hyperchromic, whilst in others heterochromia is absent. In a small proportion of cases the heterochromia is congenital. The factors determining the degree of heterochromia are the degree of atrophy of the stroma and posterior pigment layer, as well as the patient's natural iris colour. In some patients with predominantly stromal atrophy, the posterior pigmented layer shows through and becomes the dominant pigmentation so that the eye becomes hyerpchromic. In general, a brown eye becomes less brown and a blue eye assumes a more saturated blue colour.

4 Koeppe nodules are seen occasionally.

5 Rubeosis is a fairly common finding manifest as fine irregular neovascularization on the iris surface. These vessels are more fragile than normal iris vessels, and they may bleed when the pressure in the anterior chamber is suddenly reduced, as with paracentesis.

6 Enlarged pupil—atrophy of the iris sphincter may make the pupil irregular and larger than its fellow.

Vitreous   A small number of cells and stringy opacities are common.

Gonioscopy   The angle may be normal or show the following abnormalities.

Neovascularization   characterized by the presence of fine radial twig-like vessels in the chamber angle is common. These vessels are probably responsible for the filiform haemorrhages which develop with anterior chamber paracentesis 180° away from the puncture site (Amsler's sign).

Membrane   An abnormal membrane which obscures the crisp angle details may be present in the angle.

Peripheral anterior synechiae   Small, non-confluent, irregular peripheral anterior synechia are seen in some eyes.

> *Note*   Abnormal findings on gonioscopy are not necessarily related to glaucoma.

Fundus   Healed foci of choroiditis are seen in some patients and a few also have sheathing of retinal veins.

Clinical course and complications

FUS runs a chronic course lasting many years. The two main complications are cataract and glaucoma both of which may be related to the inadvertent use of topical steroids in some patients.

Cataract   This is extremely common and does not differ from that associated with other types of anterior uveitis. The results of cataract surgery are usually good, although in some cases the operation is complicated by bleeding. Short-term results of posterior-chamber intraocular lens implantation have been encouraging.

Glaucoma   This is by far the most serious threat to the patient's vision and is frequent when the

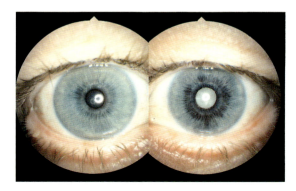

Figure 8.2 Left eye: FUS with secondary cataract. Right eye: normal eye for comparison

follow-up period is prolonged. Initially the elevation of intraocular pressure is intermittent before becoming chronic. The glaucoma is usually of the open-angle type and is thought to be caused by trabecular sclerosis. As already mentioned, fine rubeosis and peripheral anterior synechiae do not necessarily correlate with the presence of raised intraocular pressure. The glaucoma usually becomes resistant to medical therapy and filtration surgery has only a moderate degree of success.

Management

In the vast majority of cases treatment with topical steroids produces no objective improvement. Mydriatics are unnecessary as posterior synechiae do not develop. However, the patient should be examined at 4–6-monthly intervals in order to detect glaucoma.

Differential diagnosis

Intermediate uveitis Early cases of FUS may be confused with unilateral intermediate uveitis (pars planitis and chronic cyclitis) as both have cells in the anterior vitreous, relative mild anterior uveitis and absence of posterior synechiae.

Glaucomatocyclitis crisis (Posner–Schlossman syndrome) This is characterized by a mild unilateral anterior uveitis and heterochromia in about one-third of cases. However, the elevations of intraocular pressure are acute and not chronic as in FUS.

Progressive facial hemiatrophy (Parry–Romberg syndrome) This very rare condition starts in childhood and is slowly progressive. The clinical features are facial hemiatrophy which may include *en coup de sabre* (sabre stroke) on the same side as chronic iridocyclitis which may lead to iris atrophy and secondary cataract.

Intermediate uveitis

Intermediate uveitis consists of three uveitis syndromes: pars planitis, chronic cyclitis, and senile vitritis. They are all characterized by cells in the vitreous, absent or minimal anterior uveitis, and the absence of a focal fundus lesion, although some eyes have a mild peripheral retinal periphlebitis.

Pars planitis

Pars planitis accounts for about 8% of all cases of uveitis. It is an insidious chronic idiopathic intraocular inflammation which typically affects a child or a young adult.

Although both eyes are affected in about 80% of cases, the severity of involvement is frequently asymmetrical.

Symptoms

The presenting symptom is usually floaters, although occasionally the patient presents with impairment of central vision due to macular oedema. In some cases the condition is diagnosed by chance.

Signs

External The eye is invariably white.

Slitlamp The anterior chamber may be quiet or it may show a slight flare, a few cells and several small keratic precipitates. Posterior synechiae, however, are absent.

Vitreous In early cases cells are seen in the anterior vitreous. Later they assume a sheet-like configuration and small gelatinous exudates ('snowballs' or 'cotton-balls') appear (*see Figure 1.14*). Posterior vitreous detachment is common.

Pars plana and peripheral retina A mild peripheral vasculitis with sheathing of the terminal venules is common. The hallmark of pars planitis is the presence of a grey-white plaque involving the inferior pars plana (*Figure 8.3*). The plaque which is referred to as 'snowbanking' can be seen only with indirect ophthalmoscopy and scleral indentation. In advanced cases the plaque extends nasally and towards the temporal periphery as well as posteriorly to cover the peripheral retina.

Clinical course and complications

The clinical course is variable. A few patients have a single low-grade self-limiting episode lasting several months. The majority, however, have a chronic smouldering course lasting several years which may be associated with subacute exacerbations and incomplete remissions. Despite this, the visual prognosis in the majority of patients is relatively good. The three main vision threatening complications are (1) cystoid macular oedema, (2) cataract and (3) tractional retinal detachment.

Cystoid macular oedema Clinically, early macular oedema appears as a loss of the foveal reflex with a wet appearance of the posterior pole associated with many glistening highlights reflected from the irregularly thickened retina. If the oedema becomes chronic, cystoid changes develop (*Figure 8.4, left*) which may subsequently lead to a permanent impairment of visual acuity from lamellar hole formation (*Figure 8.5*).

> *Note* Fundus fluorescein angiography is helpful in detecting subtle chronic cystoid macular oedema (*Figure 8.4, right*).

Cataract As would be expected, secondary lens opacities tend to develop more frequently in eyes with severe and prolonged inflammation.

Tractional retinal detachment In advanced cases the pars plana exudate becomes vascularized from the ciliary body. The contraction of fibrovascular tissue may lead to tractional retinal detachment and vitreous haemorrhage, as well as 'dragging' of the vessels from the optic disc and heterotopia of the macula. Very rarely, a massive vascularized exudate proliferates onto the posterior lens capsule and forms a cyclitic membrane.

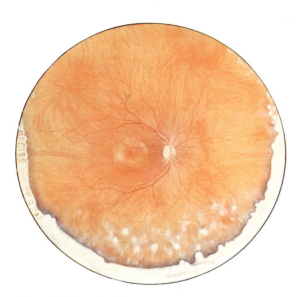

Figure 8.3 Pars planitis

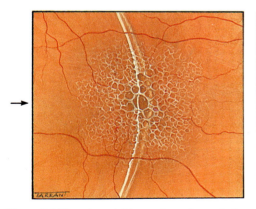
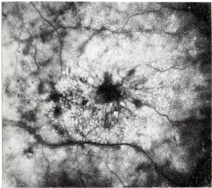

Figure 8.4 Chronic cystoid macular oedema. Left: appearance on slitlamp biomicroscopy; right: appearance of fundus fluorescein angiography (courtesy of Mr R. Whitelocke and Editor of *Transactions of the Ophthalmological Society of the UK*)

Management

It is important not to overtreat this condition. The main indication for treatment is a visual acuity of less than 6/9 due to chronic cystoid macular oedema. Most cases can be controlled and visual acuity improved by repeated posterior sub-Tenon steroid injections of methylprednisolone (Depomedrone). The necessity for repeated injections is governed by the patient's visual acuity and not the severity of vitritis. Systemic steroids can be used in the event of resistance to periocular injections. In severe steroid-resistant cases, cytotoxic agents may be of benefit (*see* Chapter 10).

Note   Topical therapy has little or no place in treatment and the benefit of cyclocryotherapy is unproven.

Differential diagnosis

Sarcoidosis   Small preretinal nodules which may resemble 'snowballs' (*see Figure 3.6*) and periphlebitis are both features of sarcoidosis. However, in most cases of sarcoidosis the anterior segment is also involved.

Toxocariasis   An inferiorly located peripheral toxocaral granuloma with a few cells in the retrolental space may be confused with pars planitis. Both conditions may also cause tractional retinal detachment as well as 'dragging' of the optic disc and heterotopia of the macula (*see Figure 5.8*). In chronic toxocaral endophthalmitis, the peripheral retina and pars plana may be covered by a dense greyish-white exudate similar to the 'snowbanking' of pars planitis. However, toxocariasis is always unilateral.

Fuchs' uveitis syndrome   Early cases of FUS with a mild anterior uveitis and cells in the anterior vitreous with absence of posterior synechiae may, on cursory examination, resemble mild unilateral pars planitis.

Birdshot chorioretinopathy   Prior to the development of the characteristic fundus lesions, the vitritis in birdshot chorioretinopathy may be mistaken for pars planitis as both are usually bilateral (*see* Chapter 9).

Candidiasis   The vitreous 'puff-balls' of ocular candidiasis (*see Figure 7.5c*) may resemble the 'snowballs' of pars planitis. However, candidiasis invariably occurs in a specific clinical setting and is associated with a multifocal retinitis.

Chronic cyclitis—clinical features

Clinically, the only difference between pars planitis and chronic cyclitis is the absence of 'snowbanking' in the latter. It has been postulated

Cystoid macular oedema

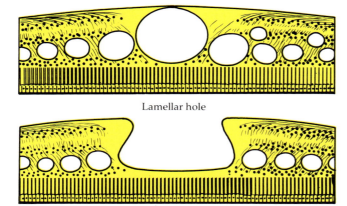

Lamellar hole

Figure 8.5 Lamellar hole formation from chronic cystoid macular oedema

that chronic cyclitis may be a forerunner or a milder form of pars planitis. Treatment is the same as for pars planitis.

Senile vitritis

This occurs in elderly patients who present with a vitritis, with absence of 'snowbanking'. In contrast to pars planitis, the cystoid macular oedema responds poorly to treatment.

Juvenile chronic iridocyclitis

Introduction

Although juvenile chronic arthritis (JCA) is the most common systemic association of chronic iridocyclitis in children, the vast majority of patients with juvenile chronic iridocyclitis are otherwise healthy. However, as in the case of chronic iridocyclitis in patients with JCA, about 75% of patients with idiopathic juvenile chronic iridocyclitis are girls.

Clinical features

Since the onset of intraocular inflammation is frequently insidious and asymptomatic, the majority of cases are not diagnosed until visual acuity is reduced from complicated cataract or the parents notice a white patch on the cornea due to band keratopathy. In a small number of cases the uveitis is detected by chance.

Signs

As in JCA—*see* Chapter 2.

Clinical course and complications

This is the same as in JCA, but the visual prognosis is less good because many eyes already have posterior synechiae, secondary cataracts or band keratopathy (*Figure 8.6*) before treatment is commenced.

Management

As for JCA.

Differential diagnosis

Juvenile chronic arthritis   In some patients with JCA the arthritis may be mild, transient and monoarticular. These patients may present with uveitis and the past history of arthritis may be overlooked by the ophthalmologist or forgotten by the patient or parents. It should also be emphasized that in about 6% of patients with JCA the uveitis antedates the arthritis by several months or even a few years.

Note   About 30% of patients with idiopathic juvenile chronic iridocyclitis are positive for antinuclear antibodies.

Intermediate uveitis   Although both pars planitis and chronic cyclitis can affect children, the anterior chamber signs are less marked and vitritis more severe than in juvenile chronic iridocyclitis. In addition, chronic cystoid macular oedema is

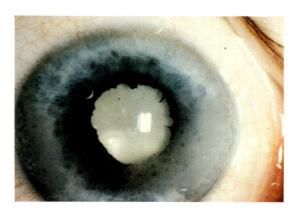

Figure 8.6 Band keratopathy and cataract in idiopathic juvenile chronic iridocyclitis

common in pars planitis but rare in juvenile chronic iridocyclitis.

> *Note* The differentiation between the two conditions is important because intermediate uveitis is treated mainly with periocular steroid injections whereas iridocyclitis usually responds to drops.

Acute anterior uveitis in young adults

Introduction

Although ankylosing spondylitis is the most common systemic association of acute anterior uveitis, many patients have no underlying systemic disease, although about 45% are carriers of HLA-B27. The risk to HLA-B27 negative patients (particularly females) of subsequently developing ankylosing spondylitis is very small, although some HLA-B27 positive patients (particularly males) will subsequently develop the disease. For this reason, patients with acute anterior uveitis who are radiologically normal, but HLA-B27 positive, should be examined at two-yearly intervals by a rheumatologist for evidence of sacro-iliac involvement.

Clinical features

As for ankylosing spondylitis—*see* Chapter 2.

Clinical course and complications

As in ankylosing spondylitis—*see* Chapter 2.

Management

See Chapter 10.

Differential diagnosis

Acute anterior uveitis in young adults also occurs in ankylosing spondylitis, Reiter's syndrome, psoriatic arthritis, sarcoidosis and Behçet's syndrome.

Further reading

Intermediate uveitis

AABERG, T.M., CESARZ, T.J. and FLICKINGER, R. (1973) Treatment of peripheral uveoretinitis by cryotherapy. *American Journal of Ophthalmology*, **75**, 685–688

CHESTER, G.H., BLACH, R.K. and CLEARY, P.E. (1976) Inflammation in the region of the vitreous base. *Transactions of the Ophthalmological Society of the United Kingdom*, **96**, 151–154

FLEDER, K.S. and BROCKHURST, R.J. (1982) Neovascular fundus abnormalities in peripheral uveitis. *Archives of Ophthalmology*, **100**, 750–754

GREEN, W.R., KINCAID, M.C., MICHELS, R.D. *et al.* (1981) Pars planitis. *Transactions of the Ophthalmological Society of the United Kingdom*, **101**, 361–367

PEDERSON, J.E., KENYON, K.R., GREEN, W.R. *et al.* (1978) Pathology of pars planitis. *American Journal of Ophthalmology*, **86**, 762–774

SMITH, R.E., GODFREY, W.A. and KIMURA, S.J. (1973) Chronic cyclitis. 1. Course and visual prognosis. *Ophthalmology*, **77**, 760–764

SMITH, R.E., GODFREY, W.A. and KIMURA, S.J. (1976) Complications of chronic cyclitis. *American Journal of Ophthalmology*, **82**, 277–282

TESSLER, H.H. (1985) What is intermediate uveitis. In *Year Book of Ophthalmology*. Ed. by J.T. Ernest. pp. 155–157. Chicago: Year Book Medical Publications

Fuchs' uveitis syndrome

ARFFA, R.C. and SCHLAEGEL, T.F. JR (1984) Chorioretinal scars in Fuchs' heterochromic iridocyclitis. *Archives of Ophthalmology*, **102**, 1153–1155

BERGER, B.B., TRESSLER, H.H. and KATTOW, M.H. (1980) Anterior segment ischaemia in Fuchs' heterochromic cyclitis. *Archives of Ophthalmology*, **98**, 499–501

KIMURA, S.J. (1978) Fuchs' syndrome of heterochromic cyclitis in brown-eyed patients. *Transactions of the American Ophthalmological Society*, **76**, 76–86

LIESEGANG, T.J. (1982) Clinical features and prognosis in Fuchs' uveitis syndrome. *Archives of Ophthalmology*, **100**, 1622–1626

MOONEY, D. and O'CONNOR, M. (1980) Intraocular lenses in Fuchs' heterochromic cyclitis. *Transactions of the Ophthalmological Society of the United Kingdom*, **100**, 510

O'CONNOR, G.R. (1985) Doyne Lecture: Heterochromic cyclitis. *Transactions of the Ophthalmological Society of the United Kingdom*, **104**, 219–231

PERRY, H.D., YANOFF, M. and SCHEIE, H.G. (1975) Rubeosis in Fuchs' heterochromic iridocyclitis. *Archives of Ophthalmology*, **93**, 337–339

SMITH, R.E. and O'CONNOR, G.R. (1974) Cataract extraction in Fuchs' syndrome. *Archives of Ophthalmology*, **91**, 39–41

WARD, D.M. and HART, C.T. (1967) Complicated cataract extraction in Fuchs' heterochromic uveitis. *British Journal of Ophthalmology*, **51**, 530–538

Juvenile chronic iridocyclitis

OHNO, S., CHAR, D.H., KIMURA, S.J. *et al.* (1977) HLA antigens and antinuclear antibody titres in juvenile chronic iridocyclitis. *British Journal of Ophthalmology,* **61**, 59–61

PERKINS, E.S. (1966) Patterns of uveitis in children. *British Journal of Ophthalmology,* **50**, 169–185

9

Rare idiopathic specific uveitis entities

Sympathetic uveitis

Introduction

Sympathetic uveitis (ophthalmitis) is a very rare, *bilateral*, granulomatous panuveitis which occurs after accidental penetrating ocular trauma (usually associated with uveal prolapse) or, less frequently, following intraocular surgery. The traumatized eye is referred to as the 'exciting eye' and the fellow eye which also develops uveitis is called the 'sympathizing eye'. Sixty-five per cent of cases of sympathetic uveitis occur between 2 weeks and 3 months after injury and 90% of cases occur within the first year.

Note It has been suggested that a single procedure, such as vitrectomy or lensectomy, is less likely to induce sympathetic uveitis than multiple attempts at secondary reconstruction of a severely traumatized eye.

Clinical features

Symptoms

The prodromal symptoms in the 'sympathizing eye' are photophobia, and blurring of vision due to loss of accommodation.

Signs

External   The 'exciting' eye shows evidence of the initial insult and is frequently excessively red and irritable.

Slitlamp   Since the inflammation starts in the ciliary body, the earliest features in the 'sympathizing eye' are cells in the retrolental space. As the inflammation becomes more severe and chronic, both eyes show Koeppe nodules, mutton fat keratic precipitates and iris thickening. Unless treated early with mydriatics, posterior synechiae form very readily.

Vitreous   A moderate to severe vitritis is present.

Fundus   Small, deep, yellow-white spots corresponding to Dalen–Fuchs' nodules are seen scattered throughout both fundi (*Figure 9.1*). Oedema

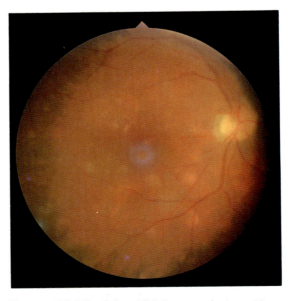

Figure 9.1 Multifocal choroiditis in sympathetic uveitis

of the optic nerve head and subretinal oedema are also frequent features.

> *Note* Very occasionally the inflammation starts in the posterior segment, but irrespective of the initial site the eventual outcome is a panuveitis.

Clinical course and complications

In a few cases the uveitis has a relatively mild and self-limited course. In the majority, however, the intraocular inflammation persists for years and may lead to cataract, glaucoma, and eventual blindness from phthisis bulbi.

> *Note* A few patients develop some of the systemic features of the Vogt–Koyanagi–Harada syndrome (*see* Chapter 3).

Management

In the vast majority of cases, enucleation (not evisceration) within two weeks of the injury will prevent sympathetic uveitis. It also seems likely that enucleation of the 'exciting' eye within two weeks of the onset of sympathetic uveitis favourably affects the eventual prognosis of the 'sympathizing' eye. The intraocular inflammation should be vigorously treated with topical, periocular and systemic steroids. Once the uveitis is controlled, steroid therapy can be gradually tapered but any acute exacerbations should be treated intensively. In severe steroid-resistant cases, cytotoxic agents, such as chlorambucil and cyclophosphamide, may be required.

Differential diagnosis

Phacoanaphylactic uveitis This, if bilateral, may be impossible to distinguish from sympathetic uveitis. However, lens extraction has a beneficial effect on the former condition but not on the latter.

> *Note* In about 20% of eyes with sympathetic uveitis a phacoanaphylactic uveitis is also present.

Vogt–Koyanagi–Harada (V-K-H) syndrome Although a few patients with sympathetic uveitis develop some of the systemic features seen in the V-K-H syndrome, a history of ocular trauma is absent in the latter, and exudative detachment of the retina, which is common in V-K-H syndrome, seldom occurs in sympathetic uveitis.

Eales' disease

Introduction

Eales' disease is an idiopathic peripheral periphlebitis which typically affects both eyes of a young male. The diagnosis should be made only after other causes of retinal periphlebitis have been excluded.

Clinical features

Symptoms

The presenting feature is usually a sudden blurring of vision due to vitreous haemorrhage.

Signs

External Nil.

Slitlamp A mild anterior uveitis may be present in some cases.

Vitreous A vitreous haze with or without blood is present.

Fundus Initially the small peripheral retinal venules show sheathing. The periphlebitis then extends more posteriorly (*Figure 9.2*) and may be associated with peripheral retinal neovascularization.

Clinical course and complications

Advanced cases are characterized by massive proliferative retinopathy with extensive retinal and vitreous haemorrhage (*Figure 9.3*) and occasionally tractional retinal detachment. Some eyes also develop rubeosis iridis, neovascular glaucoma, and cataract.

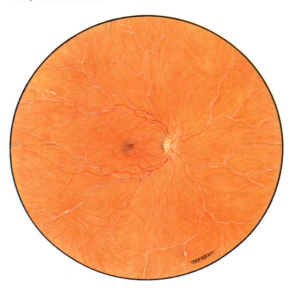

Figure 9.2 Eales' disease

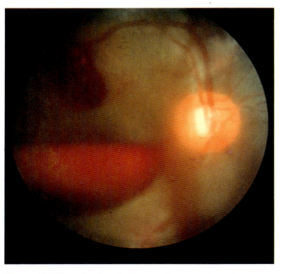

Figure 9.3 Preretinal and vitreous haemorrhage in advanced Eales' disease (courtesy of Mr P. Rosen)

Management

Treatment is unsatisfactory. In some cases, laser panretinal photocoagulation may be effective in eliminating areas of retinal ischaemia and thereby induce regression of neovascular tissue. Eyes with persistent vitreous haemorrhage or tractional retinal detachment may benefit from pars plana vitrectomy.

Differential diagnosis

Secondary periphlebitis This occurs in sarcoidosis, syphilis, pars planitis, Behçet's disease and multiple sclerosis.

Peripheral retinal neovascualrization This occurs in proliferative diabetic retinopathy, sickle-cell disease, hyperviscosity syndromes, and chronic leukaemia.

Acute posterior multifocal placoid pigment epitheliopathy

Introduction

Acute posterior multifocal placoid pigment epitheliopathy (APMPPE) is a rare idiopathic disease which typically affects both eyes of a young adult. About 50% of patients have a prodromal influenza-like illness which may be associated with erythema nodosum. The retinal pigment epithelium has been implicated as the primary site of involvement, although it has also been suggested that the disease might represent a 'vasculopathy' of the choriocapillaris.

Clinical features

Symptoms

The initial symptom is a subacute unilateral impairment of central vision. Within a few days the fellow eye usually becomes similarly involved.

Signs

External   A mild episcleral injection may be present.

Slitlamp   A few cells in the anterior chamber are common.

Vitreous   A mild vitritis is frequently present.

Fundus   The typical lesions consist of deep, placoid, cream-coloured or grey-white areas involving the postequatorial retina and posterior pole (*Figure 9.4*). A few eyes also develop vascular sheathing and disc oedema as well as serous detachment of the sensory retina. Within a few days the fellow eye shows similar changes.

Note   On fundus fluorescein angiography, the acute lesions show early blockage of background choroidal fluorescence (*Figure 9.5 left*) with late staining (*Figure 9.5 right*).

Clinical course and complications

In the vast majority of cases, the placoid lesions and vitritis resolve within a few weeks, and visual acuity returns to normal or near normal despite the presence of residual multifocal areas of depigmentation and clumping involving the retinal pigment epithelium (*Figure 9.6*). In a few cases visual acuity does not improve but recurrences do not occur.

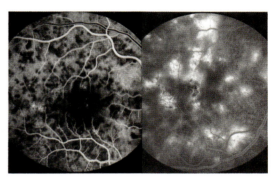

Figure 9.5 Fundus fluorescein angiogram in APMPPE. Left: early phase; right: late phase (courtesy of Professor A. Bird)

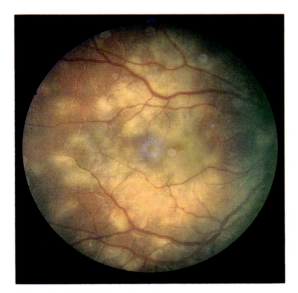

Figure 9.4 APMPPE: active stage

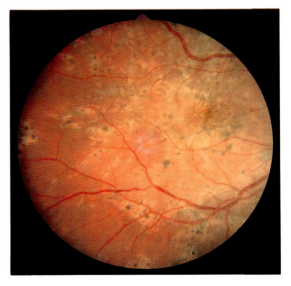

Figure 9.6 Changes in retinal pigment epithelium following resolution of APMPPE

> *Note*   During the inactive healed stage, fundus fluorescein angiography shows increased background choroidal fluorescein due to retinal pigment epithelial 'window' defects but no staining.

Management

There is no effective treatment.

Serpiginous choroidopathy

Introduction

Serpiginous (geographical) choroidopathy is a rare, idiopathic, recurrent disease of the retinal pigment epithelium and choriocapillaris which typically affects patients between the fourth and sixth decades of life. Involvement is bilateral although its extent is frequently asymmetrical.

Signs

External   Nil.

Slitlamp   A mild anterior uveitis is seen occasionally.

Vitreous   A vitritis is present in some eyes.

Clinical features

Symptoms

The patient is asymptomatic unless the fovea is involved.

Fundus   The chorioretinal lesions usually start around the optic disc (*Figure 9.7*) and spread outwards in all directions. The acute lesions consist of cream-coloured opacities with hazy borders at the level of the retinal pigment epithelium. They persist for a few weeks, eventually becoming lighter in colour, and over the subsequent months they become inactive, leaving scalloped 'punched out' areas of retinal pigment epithelial and choroidal atrophy. Large choroidal blood vessels in the base of an area of atrophy

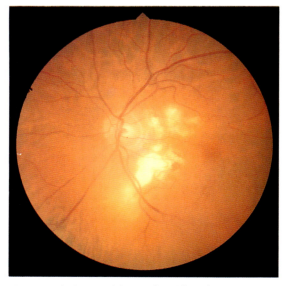

Figure 9.7 Active serpiginous choroidopathy

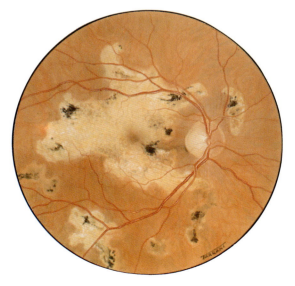

Figure 9.8 Advanced serpiginous choroidopathy

frequently are the only visible remnants of the choroid (*Figure 9.8*). Fresh acute lesions then usually arise as extensions from old inactive scars.

> *Note* On fundus fluorescein angiography, the acute lesions show early blockage of background choroidal fluorescence with late staining.

Clinical course and complications

Successive attacks result in pseudopodal extension of the destructive process peripherally from the peripapillary area in an irregular, convoluted, snake-like manner. Involvement of the fovea causes a profound and permanent impairment of central vision (*Figure 9.9*). Eyes in which the fovea is bypassed are not always safe from future foveal involvement, as occasionally the lesions begin in an extrapapillary location and subsequently spread centrally towards the optic disc. Subretinal neovascularization occurs in some cases.

> *Note* On fundus fluorescein angiography, the old inactive lesions show early hypofluorescence due to decreased background choroidal fluorescence from atrophy of the choriocapillaris (*Figure 9.10 left*). However, later there is hyperfluorescence at the margins of the atrophic areas due to diffusion of dye from the bordering normal choriocapillaris (*Figure 9.10 right*) and, in very late pictures, the atrophic areas themselves are diffusely hyperfluorescent as the dye stains the sclera and fibrous tissue.

Management

There is no effective treatment

Differential diagnosis

APMPPE Although the active lesions of APMPPE and serpiginous choroidopathy have similar fundoscopic and angiographic appearances, the former occurs in younger individuals and has a more acute course with a much better visual prognosis. In APMPPE, the new lesions tend to arise independently, whereas in serpiginous choroidopathy new lesions arise predominantly as extensions from pre-existing scars.

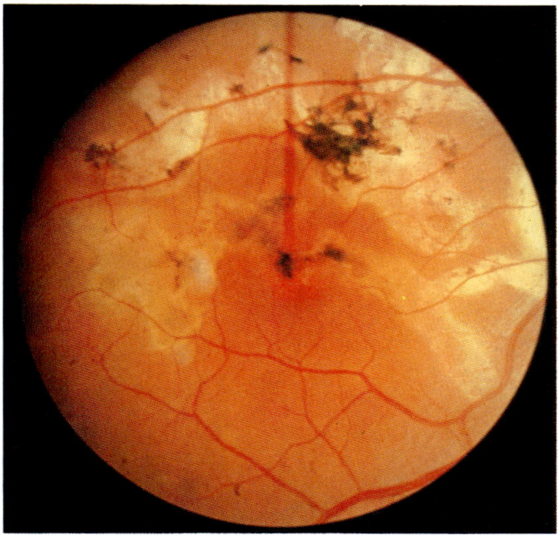

Figure 9.9 Involvement of fovea by serpiginous choroidopathy (courtesy of Professor A. Bird)

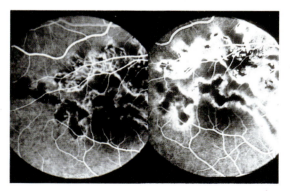

Figure 9.10 Fundus fluorecein angiogram in serpiginous choroidopathy. Left: early phase; right: late phase (courtesy of Professor A. Bird)

Birdshot retinochoroidopathy

Introduction

Birdshot retinochoroidopathy (vitiliginous retinochoroiditis) is a very rare, idiopathic, bilateral, chronic, multifocal choroidopathy and vasculopathy. It typically affects healthy middle-aged individuals who are positive for HLA-A29 and is more common in women than in men.

Clinical features

Symptoms

The initial symptoms are either vitreous floaters or, less commonly, blurring of central vision due to macular oedema.

Signs

External   The eye is invariably white.

Slitlamp   A mild anterior uveitis with small to medium-sized keratic precipitates may be present.

Vitreous   A diffuse vitritis is present with the cellular infiltration most dense posteriorly.

> *Note*   Vitreous 'snowballs' and 'snowbanking' are absent.

Fundus   The postequatorial regions of both fundi show varying numbers of flat creamy-yellow spots due to focal hypopigmentation of the choroid and retinal pigment epithelium (*Figure 9.11*). The diameter of each lesion is between half to one disc and their borders are not sharply demarcated. The retinal vessels are undisturbed as they pass over the lesions and the larger choroidal vessels can be seen within each individual lesion (*Figure 9.12*). Although initially the spots do not involve the macula, later they may become more confluent and spread to the macula. After a few weeks or months, the individual spots evolve into more atrophic white depigmented lesions which are more circumscribed but which are not associated with secondary hyperpigmentation.

Occasionally, the peripheral retinal blood vessels show sheathing and some eyes have disc oedema.

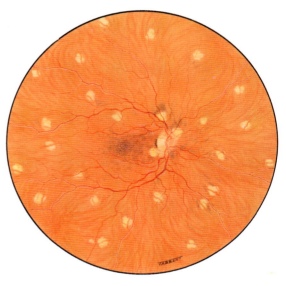

Figure 9.11 Birdshot retinochoroidopathy

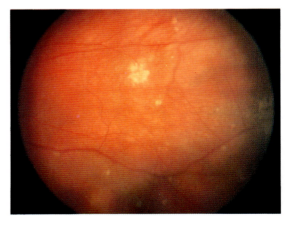

Figure 9.12 Birdshot retinochoroidopathy (courtesy of Dr J. Federman)

ERG may show an abnormal scotopic and photopic response with decreased amplitude and delay in latency.

Clinical course and complications

The disease runs a chronic course lasting several years with remissions and exacerbations with eventual stabilization and retention of useful vision in at least one eye. The main causes of visual impairment are: (1) chronic cystoid macular oedema, (2) geographical atrophy of macula, (3) serous detachment of sensory retina, (4) secondary cataract, (5) optic atrophy and, occasionally, (6) subretinal neovascularization.

Management

Topical, periocular and systemic steroids have been tried but have not been found to be beneficial.

Differential diagnosis

Intermediate uveitis Prior to the development of the characteristic fundus lesions, the vitritis in patients with birdshot retinochoroidopathy may be mistaken for chronic cyclitis or pars planitis. Senile vitritis, however, occurs in older individuals than birdshot retinochoroidopathy.

APMPPE The fundus lesions of birdshot retinochoroidopathy may be confused with APMPPE. However, the latter disorder has a rapid course and resolution whereas the former has a more chronic and relentless course.

Acute retinal necrosis

Introduction

Acute retinal necrosis (ARN) is an extremely rare but devastating necrotizing retinitis. It affects otherwise healthy individuals of all ages and is bilateral in 30–50% of cases. The herpes zoster virus has been isolated from the retina in a few cases and may be the causative agent.

Clinical features

Symptoms

The initial symptoms are periorbital pain followed by blurring of vision.

Signs

External Diffuse episcleral injection may be present.

Slitlamp An anterior uveitis with small or 'mutton fat' keratic precipitates usually precedes the posterior segment changes,

Vitreous This shows cellular infiltration.

Fundus The initial findings may involve either the posterior pole or the fundus periphery. The retinal arterioles appear sheathed and deep, multifocal, yellow-white patches begin to appear within the retina. The lesions, which may be associated with retinal haemorrhages, gradually become confluent and represent a full-thickness necrotizing retinitis. In cases that start in the periphery, the posterior fundus central to the vascular arcades is spared so that visual acuity may remain fairly good despite severe necrosis of the surrounding retina (*Figure 9.13a*).

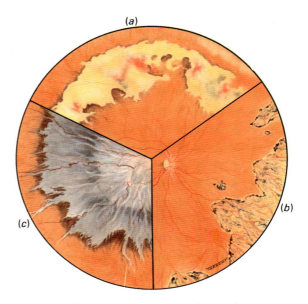

Figure 9.13 Progression of acute retinal necrosis

Clinical course and complications

The acute retinitis resolves within 4–12 weeks leaving behind transparent and necrotic retina with atrophy of the retinal pigment epithelium (*Figure 9.13b*). About 70% of eyes develop retinal holes, usually at the margin of uninvolved and involved zones, which lead to rhegmatogenous retinal detachment (*Figure 9.13c*). In some eyes, secondary vitreous fibrosis gives rise to tractional retinal detachments. In both instances, the retinal detachment is extremely difficult to repair due to the development of gross proliferative vitreoretinopathy.

Management

Treatment with antibiotics, steroids and cytotoxic agents has been tried, but found to be ineffective.

Differential diagnosis

CMV retinitis   Although ARN may resemble CMV retinitis, the latter is usually associated with more haemorrhage and spreads more slowly. In addition patients with ARN are immunologically normal.

Behçet's disease   In Behçet's disease the retinal changes are also caused by vasculitis and infarction (*see* Chapter 3). However, the course of ARN is usually more rapid and patients are otherwise healthy.

Multifocal choroiditis with progressive subretinal fibrosis

Introduction

This recently described idiopathic specific uveitis entity typically affects both eyes of young, otherwise healthy, females.

Clinical features

Symptoms

The initial symptom is an abrupt onset of visual loss in one or both eyes.

Signs

External   Nil.

Slitlamp   A mild anterior uveitis is frequently present.

Vitreous   Most eyes have a mild vitritis.

Fundus   The initial findings consist of clusters of small hypopigmented choroidal lesions scattered throughout the posterior pole and mid-retinal periphery. Within two to four weeks the acute lesions heal with the formation of stellate subretinal scars.

Clinical course and complications

During the course of the disease, serous and haemorrhagic detachments of the macula may develop in some patients. After several months, the subretinal scars enlarge and coalesce to form large zones of subretinal fibrosis with irregular borders (*Figure 9.14*). Involvement of the macula causes a profound and permanent loss of central vision.

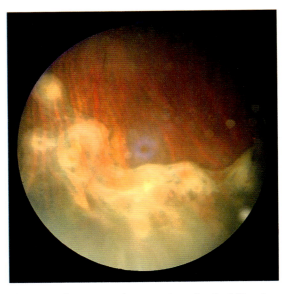

Figure 9.14 Late stage of progressive subretinal fibrosis

Management

The acute stage of the disease may respond to systemic steroid therapy, but once the subretinal scars have formed treatment is ineffective.

Differential diagnosis

Although the acute multifocal lesions may be mistaken for APMPPE or birdshot retinochoroidopathy, the subretinal fibrosis is unique to this disease.

Glaucomatocyclitic crisis

Introduction

Glaucomatocyclitic crisis (Posner–Schlossman syndrome) is characterized by recurrent attacks of secondary open-angle glaucoma with mild anterior uveitis. The disease typically affects young adults, 40% of whom are positive for HLA-Bw54. During an attack, the intraocular pressure is usually severely elevated (40–60 mmHg) for between a few hours to several days. The attacks are unilateral, although 50% of patients have bilateral involvement at different times.

Clinical features

Symptoms

Haloes around lights are frequent during an acute attack, although pain is rare.

Signs

External The eye is invariably white.

Slitlamp Epithelial oedema may be present but the anterior chamber is not shallow. The aqueous contains a few cells but no flare. A few fine non-pigmented keratic precipitates are also present, but posterior synechiae do not develop.

Vitreous A few cells are present in the anterior vitreous.

Fundus The fundus is normal.

Clinical course and complications

Although the intervals between attacks vary in length, with the passage of time they usually become longer and, in rare cases, a chronic rise in intraocular pressure develops. This may lead to cupping of the optic disc and loss of visual field. Some patients develop a mild heterochromia.

Management

During an attack, the intraocular pressure can be reduced medically and surgical intervention is rarely necessary. The beneficial effect of topical steroids is doubtful.

Differential diagnosis

Primary angle-closure glaucoma A history of intermittent haloes and the presence of corneal oedema may lead to the misdiagnosis of acute or subacute primary angle-closure glaucoma. However, in glaucomatocyclitic crisis, the anterior chamber is usually of normal depth and gonioscopy shows an open angle. Patients with primary angle-closure glaucoma are also usually older.

Fuchs' uveitis syndrome Both conditions may be associated with elevation of intraocular pressure, absence of posterior synechiae and heterochromia. However, in FUS the keratic precipitates are characteristic and the patient does not complain of haloes as the rise of intraocular pressure is usually chronic and not acute.

Further reading

Sympathetic uveitis
BLODI, F.C. (1979) Sympathetic uveitis. In *Ocular Trauma*. Ed. by H.M. Freeman. pp. 417–427. New York: Appleton-Century-Crofts
BRAUNINGER, G.E. and POLACK, F.M. (1971) Sympathetic ophthalmitis. *American Journal of Ophthalmology*, **72**, 967–968
LEWIS, M.L., GASS, J.D.M. and SPENCER, W.H. (1978) Sympathetic uveitis after trauma and vitrectomy. *Archives of Ophthalmology*, **96**, 263–267
LUBIN, J.R., ALBERT, D.M. and WEINSTEIN, M. (1980) Sixty-five years of sympathetic ophthalmia: a clinicopathologic review of 105 cases (1913–1978). *Ophthalmology*, **87**, 109–121
MACKLEY, T.A. and AZAR, A. (1978) Sympathetic ophthalmia: a long-term follow-up. *Archives of Ophthalmology*, **96**, 257–262

McPHERSON, S.D.JR and DALTON, H.T. (1975) Posterior form of sympathetic ophthalmia. *Transactions of the American Ophthalmological Society*, **73**, 251–263

MARAK, G.E. (1979) Recent advances in sympathetic ophthalmia. *Survey of Ophthalmology*, **24**, 141–156

RAO, N.A., ROBIN, J., DARTMAN, S. *et al.* (1983) The role of penetrating wound in the development of sympathetic ophthalmia—experimental observations. *Archives of Ophthalmology*, **101**, 102–104

RAO, N.A. and WONG, V.G. (1981) Aetiology of sympathetic ophthalmitis. *Transactions of the Ophthalmological Society of the United Kingdom*, **101**, 357–360

Acute posterior multifocal placoid pigment epitheliopathy

DAMATO, B.E., NANJIANI, M. and FOULDS, W.S. (1983) Acute posterior multifocal placoid pigment epitheliopathy. A follow-up study. *Transactions of the Ophthalmological Society of the United Kingdom*, **103**, 517–522

FISHMAN, G.B., RAAB, M.F. and KAPLAN, J. (1974) Acute posterior multifocal placoid pigment epitheliopathy. *Archives of Ophthalmology*, **92**, 173–177

FITZPATRICK, P.J., ROBERTSON, D.M. and ROCHESTER, M.N. (1973) Acute posterior multifocal placoid pigment epitheliopathy. *Archives of Ophthalmology*, **89**, 373–376

GASS, J.D.M. (1968) Acute posterior multifocal placoid pigment epitheliopathy. *Archives of Ophthalmology*, **80**, 177–185

HOLT, W.S., REGAN, C.D.J. and TREMPE, C. (1976) Acute posterior multifocal placoid pigment epitheliopathy. *American Journal of Ophthalmology*, **81**, 403–412

KIRKHAM, T.H., FFYTCHE, T.J. and SANDERS, M.D. (1972) Placoid pigment epitheliopathy with retinal vasculitis and papillitis. *British Journal of Ophthalmology*, **56**, 875–880

LEWIS, R.A. and MARTONYI, C.L. (1975) Acute posterior multifocal placoid pigment epitheliopathy. A recurrence. *Archives of Ophthalmology*, **93**, 235–238

MURRAY, S.B. (1979) Acute posterior multifocal placoid pigment epitheliopathy. Not so benign? *Transactions of the Ophthalmological Society of the United Kingdom*, **99**, 497–500

RYAN, S.J. and MAUMENEE, A.E. (1972) Acute posterior multifocal placoid pigment epitheliopathy. *American Journal of Ophthalmology*, **74**, 1066–1074

SAVINO, P.J., WEINBERG, R.J., YASSIN, J.G. *et al.* (1974) Diverse manifestations of acute posterior multifocal placoid pigment epitheliopathy. *American Journal of Ophthalmology*, **77**, 659–662

Serpiginous choroidopathy

CHISHOLM, I.H., GASS, J.D.M. and HUTTON, W.L. (1976) The late stage of serpiginous (geographic) choroiditis. *American Journal of Ophthalmology*, **82**, 343–351

HAMILTON, A.M. and BIRD, A.C. (1974) Geographical choroidopathy. *British Journal of Ophthalmology*, **58**, 784–797

LAATIKAINEN, L. and ERKKILA, H. (1974) Serpiginous choroiditis. *British Journal of Ophthalmology*, **58**, 777–783

Birdshot retinochoroidopathy

FREUST, D.J., TRESSLER, H.H., FISHMAN, G.A. *et al.* (1984) Birdshot retinochoroidopathy. *Archives of Ophthalmology*, **102**, 214–219

GASS, J.D.M. (1981) Vitiliginous chorioretinitis. *Archives of Ophthalmology*, **99**, 1778–1787

KAPLAN, H.J. and AABERG, T.M. (1980) Birdshot retinochoroidopathy. *American Journal of Ophthalmology*, **90**, 773–782

NUSSENBLATT, R.B., MITTAL, K.K., RYAN, S. *et al.* (1982) Birdshot choroidopathy associated with HLA-A29 antigen and immune responsiveness to retinal S-antigen. *American Journal of Ophthalmology*, **94**, 147–158

RYAN, S.J. and MAUMENEE, A.E. (1980) Birdshot retinochoroidopathy. *American Journal of Ophthalmology*, **89**, 31–45

Acute retinal necrosis

CULBERTSON, W.W., BLUMENKRANZ, M., HAINES, H. *et al.* (1982) Acute retinal necrosis syndrome. Part 2. Histopathology and etiology. *Ophthalmology*, **89**, 1317–1324

CULBERTSON, W.W., CLARKSON, J.G., BLUMENKRANZ, M.S. *et al.* (EDITORIAL) (1983) Acute retinal necrosis. *American Journal of Ophthalmology*, **96**, 683–685

FISHER, J.P., LEWIS, M.L., BLUMENKRANZ, M. *et al.* (1982) The acute retinal necrosis syndrome. Part 1. Clinical manifestations. *Ophthalmology*, **89**, 1309–1316

GORMAN, B.D., NADEL, A.J. and COLES, R.S. (1982) Acute retinal necrosis. *Ophthalmology*, **89**, 809–814

PRICE, F.W. JR and SCHLAEGEL, T.F. JR (1980) Bilateral acute retinal necrosis. *American Journal of Ophthalmology*, **89**, 419–424

SAARI, K.M., BOKE, W., MANTHEY, K.F. *et al.* (1982) Bilateral acute retinal necrosis. *American Journal of Ophthalmology*, **93**, 403–411

YOUNG, N.J.A. and BIRD, A.C. (1978) Bilateral acute retinal necrosis. *British Journal of Ophthalmology*, **62**, 581–590

Multifocal choroiditis with progressive subretinal fibrosis

CANTRILL, H.L. and FOLK, J.C. (1986) Multifocal choroiditis associated with progressive subretinal fibrosis. *American Journal of Ophthalmology*, **101**, 170–180

DORAN, R. and HAMILTON, A. (1982) Disciform macular degeneration in young adults. *Transactions of the Ophthalmological Society of the United Kingdom*, **102**, 471–480

PALESTINE, A., NUSSENBLATT, R., PARVER, L. and KNOX, D. (1984) Progressive subretinal fibrosis and uveitis. *British Journal of Ophthalmology*, **68**, 667–673

Glaucomatocyclitic crisis

HIROSE, S., OHNO, S. and MATSUDA, H. (1985) HLA-Bw54 and glaucomatocyclitic crisis. *Archives of Ophthalmology*, **103**, 1837–1839

KASS, M.A., BECKER, B. and KOLKER, A.E. (1973) Glaucomatocyclitic crisis and primary open-angle glaucoma. *American Journal of Ophthalmology*, **75**, 668–673

RAITTA, C. and VANNAS, A. (1977) Glaucomatocyclitic crisis. *Archives of Ophthalmology*, **95**, 608–612

10

Management of uveitis

Aims of therapy

The three main aims of treating uveitis are:

1 To prevent vision threatening complications, such as glaucoma, cataract, chronic cystoid macular oedema, and retinal detachment.
2 To relieve the patient's discomfort.
3 To treat the underlying cause if possible.

The four main groups of drugs used in the treatment of uveitis are mydriatics, steroids, cytotoxic agents, and cyclosporin. Patients with uveitis caused by infections should be treated with the appropriate antimicrobial or antiviral agent.

Mydriatics

In *Table 10.1* are shown the properties of the main topical mydriatics used in the management of uveitis.

Indications

Mydriatics are used for three reasons.

To give comfort   The discomfort caused by severe acute anterior uveitis is due to spasm of the ciliary muscle and the sphincter of the pupil. This can be relieved by using atropine which is the most powerful cycloplegic available. It is usually unnecessary to use atropine for more than one or two weeks. Once the inflammation is showing signs of subsiding it can be substituted by a short-acting mydriatic, such as tropicamide or cyclopentolate.

To prevent posterior synechiae   This is best achieved by using a short-acting mydriatic which keeps the pupil mobile. In mild cases of chronic anterior uveitis the mydriatic can be instilled once a day at bedtime to prevent difficulties with accommodation during the day. In eyes with chronic anterior uveitis, the pupil should not be kept constantly dilated as posterior synechiae can still form in the dilated position. In young

Table 10.1 Topical mydriatics used in uveitis

Drug	Mydriasis		Cycloplegia	
	Maximal effect (min)	Full recovery (days)	Maximal effect (h)	Full recovery (days)
Atropine 1%	40	10+	6	14
Hyoscine (0.25% and 0.5%) (scopolamine)	30	7	1	7
Homatropine (1%–5%)	60	3	1	3
Cyclopentolate (0.5%–2%) (Mydrilate, Cyclogyl)	60	1	1	1
Tropicamide (0.5% and 1%) (Mydriacyl)	40	0.25	0.5	0.25
Phenylephrine 10% (Neosynephrine)	20	0.25	Nil	—

The values given are for the strongest concentrations.

children, constant atropinization of one eye may induce amblyopia.

Note Do not use mydriatics in FUS because posterior synechiae never form.

To break down synechiae The formation of posterior synechiae is undesirable as it interferes with the normal action of the pupil, it may cause pupil block glaucoma due to seclusio pupillae, and also promotes the development of complicated cataract. Once significant synechiae have formed, intensive topical mydriatic therapy with atropine, phenylephrine, and cocaine is seldom effective in breaking them down, although an anterior sub-Tenon's injection of Mydricaine (adrenaline, atropine and procaine) may be effective if the synechiae are new and unassociated with fibrosis.

Steroids

Steroids are still the mainstay in the management of most cases of uveitis. They can be administered topically in the form of drops or ointment, by periocular injection, or systemically.

Topical administration

Preparations

In *Table 10.2* are shown the main topical steroid preparations (available in the UK) in decreasing order of anti-inflammatory power.

Table 10.2 Topical steroids used in uveitis

Generic name	Drops	Ointment
Dexamethasone 0.1% (Maxidex)	+	
Betamethasone sodium phosphate 0.1% (Betnesol)	+	+
Prednisolone sodium phosphate 0.5% (Predsol)	+	
Fluorometholone 0.1% (FML)	+	
Clobetasone butyrate 0.1% (Eumovate)	+	

Severe forms of anterior uveitis can be treated with the powerful steroids, such as dexamethasone, betamethasone, and prednisolone, whilst the weaker preparations such as fluorometholone and clobetasone are reserved for relatively mild uveitis in patients who are steroid reactors. This is because the latter two drugs have a lesser propensity to elevate intraocular pressure in susceptible individuals than the more powerful preparations.

Note A solution penetrates the cornea better than a suspension or ointment. Ointment can, however, be instilled before going to bed.

Indications

Topical steroids can only be used in the treatment of anterior uveitis because they cannot reach a therapeutic level in tissues that are behind the lens.

Frequency of instillation

The frequency of instillation of drops depends on the severity of inflammation and can vary from one drop every five minutes to one drop every other day. In general, one should start with a high rate of instillation and then decrease as the inflammation lessens, rather than start with a low rate and work up. This principle applies to both topical and systemic administration of steroids. The management of acute anterior uveitis is relatively straightforward and treatment can usually be tapered after a few days and then discontinued after five to six weeks. The treatment of chronic anterior uveitis is very much more difficult because steroid therapy may have to be given for many months and even years. In these cases, acute exacerbations with +4 aqueous cells are treated with hourly instillation for two to three days and then the drops are tapered to four times a day. If the inflammation is under good control with no more than +1 aqueous cells, then the rate of instillation can be further reduced gradually over the next few months and then stopped. Following cessation of drops, the patient should be re-examined within a few days to ensure that the uveitis has not recurred.

Complications

The following complications may occur from topical steroid administration.

Glaucoma The application of a potent steroid four times a day for six weeks will cause a marked elevation of intraocular pressure (to over 31 mmHg) in about 5% of the general population. A further 35% show a moderate rise (between 22 and 30 mmHg) and the remaining 60% show virtually no change. The stronger steroids, such as dexamethasone, betamethasone, and prednisolone, are probably equipotent in their ability to raise intraocular pressure but weaker steroids, such as fluorometholone and clobetasone, have a low propensity for elevating intraocular pressure.

Cataract Posterior subcapsular cataract can be promoted by both systemic and, less frequently, topical steroid administration. The risk increases with the amount and duration of therapy.

Corneal complications These are as follows:
1 Reduction of immunological protection against secondary infection with bacteria and fungi.
2 Enhancement of recrudescences and multiplication of HSV.
3 Corneal melting may be enhanced due to the inhibition of collagen synthesis.

Systemic absorption Systemic side-effects may be induced following prolonged administration, particularly in children.

Mydriasis and ptosis These are transient and reversible and may be caused by the preservative and not the steroid.

Periocular injections

Preparations

In *Table 10.3* are shown the four main steroids available for periocular injection.

Table 10.3 Main steroids used for periocular injections

Short-acting (1 day)	Long-acting (several weeks)
Betamethasone 4 mg/ml	Methylprednisolone acetate 40 mg/ml
Dexamethasone 4 mg/ml	Triamcinolone acetonide 40 mg/ml

Advantages over drops

Periocular injections have the following advantages:
1 They are able to reach a therapeutic concentration behind the lens.
2 Drugs that are only water soluble and incapable of penetrating the cornea when given topically can enter the eye by penetrating the sclera when given by periocular injection.
3 A long-lasting effect can be achieved if a depot preparation such as methylprednisolone (Depomedrone) is used.

Indications

1 Severe acute anterior uveitis, especially in patients with ankylosing spondylitis with a marked fibrinous exudate in the anterior chamber (*see Figure 2.2*) or hypopyon.
2 As an adjunct to topical or systemic therapy in resistant cases of chronic anterior uveitis.
2 Intermediate uveitis.
4 Poor patient compliance.
5 At the time of surgery in eyes with uveitis.

Techniques of administration

Periocular injections can be subconjunctival, anterior sub-Tenon, posterior sub-Tenon, and retrobulbar. Subconjunctival injections are given mainly for the treatment of corneal inflammations and retrobulbar injections are now seldom used. For these reasons, only the two types of sub-Tenon's injections will be described.

Preparation of patient It is extremely important to have the conjunctiva very well anaesthetized prior to attempting a periocular injection. If this is done correctly, the injection can be given with minimal discomfort to the patient. The conjunctiva is anaesthetized as follows:
1 Instill a topical anaesthetic such as amethocaine or cocaine at 1-min intervals tor 10 min.
2 Place a small cotton pledget impregnated with cocaine into the conjunctival sac at the site of injection (*Figure 10.1 top*) and leave it there for 5 min (*Figure 10.1 bottom*).

Anterior sub-Tenon injection technique

1 Draw up 1 ml of steroid into a 2-ml syringe and replace the drawing up needle with a number 25 gauge 3/8 inch (10 mm) disposable needle.
2 Ask the patient to look away from the site of injection.
3 With toothed (St Martin's) forceps grasp conjunctiva and Tenon's.
4 With the bevel away from the eye, pass the needle through conjunctiva and Tenon's at the point where they are grasped.
5 Slowly inject 0.5 ml of steroid.

Note   Anterior sub-Tenon's injections are used mainly in the treatment of severe or resistant anterior uveitis.

Posterior sub-Tenon injection technique

1 Draw up 1.5 ml of steroid into a 2-ml syringe (*Figure 10.2 left*) and replace the drawing up needle with a number 25 gauge 5/8 inch (16 mm) disposable needle (*Figure 10.2 right*).
2 Ask the patient to look away from the site of injection which is usually in the upper or lower temporal quadrant.
3 Evert the eyelid and penetrate the bulbar conjunctiva with the tip of the needle (bevel towards the globe) slightly on the global side of the fornix (*Figure 10.3*).
4 Slowly insert the needle posteriorly keeping it as close to the globe as possible.

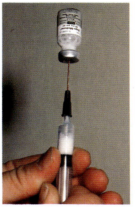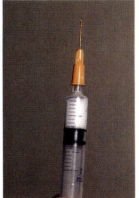

Figure 10.2 Left: drawing up of methylprednisolone (Depomedrone); right: 25 gauge, 5/8 inch needle for posterior sub-Tenon injection

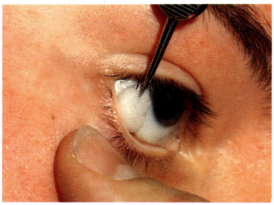
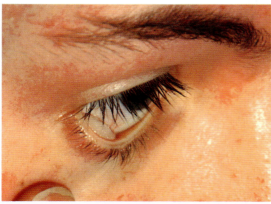

Figure 10.1 Top: insertion of cotton pledget into inferior fornix; bottom: pledget *in situ*

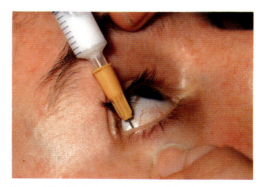

Figure 10.3 Posterior sub-Tenon injection

Note In order not to penetrate the globe accidentally with the tip of the needle make wide side-to-side motions as you are inserting the needle and watch the limbus—movement of the limbus means that you have engaged the sclera!

5 When the needle cannot be inserted any further withdraw the plunger slightly and if no blood has entered the syringe inject 1 ml of steroid.

Note If the needle is too far away from the globe, adequate trans-scleral absorption of the steroid will not occur. The posterior sub-Tenon injection is indicated for intermediate uveitis and as an alternative to systemic therapy of posterior uveitis.

Systemic therapy

Preparations

The main oral preparation for systemic use is prednisolone 5 mg. Enteric coated (2.5 mg) tablets can be used in patients with a history of gastric ulceration. Injections of adrenocorticotropic hormone (ACTH) can be used in the few patients who are intolerant to oral therapy.

Indications

The main indications for systemic therapy are:
1 Intractable anterior uveitis which has failed to respond to both topical therapy and anterior sub-Tenon injections.
2 Intractable intermediate uveitis which has failed to respond to posterior sub-Tenon injections.
3 Posterior uveitis which has failed to respond to posterior sub-Tenon injections.

Rules in the use of systemic steroids

1 Start with a large dose and then reduce.

2 The initial daily dose of prednisolone is 1–1.5 mg/kg body weight.
3 The total dose should be taken before eating breakfast.
4 Switch to an every-other-breakfast regimen once the inflammation is brought under control and then taper gradually over several weeks.
5 If steroids are given for less than 2 weeks there is no need to reduce the dose gradually.

Side-effects

Short steroid therapy
1 Peptic ulceration.
2 Mental changes.
3 Aseptic necrosis of the head of the femur.
4 Hyperosmolar hyperglycaemic non-ketotic coma (very rare).

Long steroid therapy
1 Osteoporosis.
2 Cushingoid state (*Figure 10.4*).
3 Electrolyte imbalance.
4 Reactivation of infections, such as TB.
5 Cataract.
6 Increase in severity of pre-existing disease, such as diabetes.
7 Limitation of growth in children (*Figure 10.4*).
8 Myopathy.

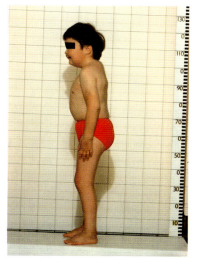

Figure 10.4 Cushingoid state and stunted growth in a boy due to systemic steroids (courtesy of Dr B. Ansell)

When not to use steroids

1 In inactive disease with a chronic flare but no cells.
2 In mild anterior uveitis with not more than a +1 cell.
3 In intermediate uveitis with normal vision.
4 In Fuchs' uveitis syndrome.
5 When antimicrobial therapy is more appropriate, e.g. candidiasis.

Cytotoxic agents

Introduction

Cytotoxic agents are drugs which were initially used for the treatment of certain malignant diseases. The three main groups that have been used in the treatment of uveitis are shown in *Table 10.4*.

Table 10.4 Main groups of cytotoxic agents used in uveitis

Group	Drugs
Antifoliates	Methotrexate
Antipurines	6-Mercaptopurine Azathioprine
Alkylating agents	Chlorambucil Cyclophosphamide

Since all of these drugs are potentially toxic, their administration should be supervised by a physician. Complications of cytotoxic drugs include: bone marrow depression, gastrointestinal ulceration, stomatitis, liver damage, sterility, alopecia, neoplasia, haemorrhagic cystitis, genetic damage, and nausea and vomiting. Methotrexate and 6-mercaptopurine are now seldom used because of their relatively serious side-effects and poor results in the treatment of uveitis.

Indications

The two main general indications for the use of cytotoxic agents are:

1 Potentially binding (usually bilateral) reversible intraocular inflammation which has failed to respond to *adequate* steroid therapy.

2 Intolerable side-effects from systemic steroid therapy.

Specific types of uveitis that have been treated with cytotoxic agents include the following.

Behçet's disease Due to the poor visual prognosis, posterior uveitis associated with Behçet's disease is considered by many to be an absolute indication for cytotoxic agents. The most commonly used drug is chlorambucil. In about 50% of patients, the intraocular inflammation is stabilized, and in 25% it is improved. The remainder continue to deteriorate.

Sympathetic uveitis This is probably only a relative indication for cytotoxic drugs, since the majority of cases can be controlled by adequate steroid therapy. Both chlorambucil and cyclophosphamide have been found to be beneficial in steroid-resistant cases.

Intermediate uveitis This is a very rare indication as most cases can be controlled by periocular steroid injections. In severe intractable cases, azathioprine, chlorambucil, and cyclophosphamide may be beneficial.

Juvenile chronic arthritis The results of treatment of intractable uveitis with chlorambucil have been equivocal.

Note So far no double-blind controlled trial of cytotoxic therapy for uveitis has been published.

Cyclosporin

Cyclosporin is a powerful anti-T-cell immunosuppressive agent. Preliminary uncontrolled studies have shown that it is a promising agent in the treatment of steroid and/or cytotoxic resistant cases of Behçet's uveitis, intermediate uveitis, sympathetic uveitis, and sarcoid uveitis. Unfortunately, an unacceptable high rate of renal toxicity makes it an unacceptable drug for routine use.

Further reading

Management of uveitis

DINNING, W.J. (1981) Treatment of uveitis. *Transactions of the Ophthalmological Society of the United Kingdom,* **101**, 391–393

DINNING, W.J. (1983) Therapy—selected topics. In *Uveitis, Pathophysiology and Therapy.* Eds E. Kraus-Mackiw and G.R. O'Connor. pp. 198–220. New York: Thieme-Stratton Inc.

DINNING, W.J. and PERKINS, E.S. (1975) Immunosuppressives in uveitis. A preliminary report of experience with chlorambucil. *British Journal of Ophthalmology,* **59**, 397–403

GODFREY, W.A., EPSTEIN, W.V., O'CONNOR, G.R. *et al.* (1974) Use of chlorambucil in intractable idiopathic uveitis. *American Journal of Ophthalmology,* **78**, 415–428

GRAHAM, E.M., SANDERS, M.D., JAMES, D.G. *et al.* (1985) Cyclosporin A in the treatment of posterior uveitis. *British Journal of Ophthalmology,* **104**, 146–151

MEHRA, R., MOORE, T.L., CATALANO, J.D. *et al.* (1981) Chlorambucil in the treatment of iridocyclitis in juvenile rheumatoid arthritis. *Journal of Rheumatology,* **8**, 141–144

NUSSENBLATT, R.B., PALESTINE, A.G. and CHAN, C.C. (1983) Cyclosporin A in the treatment of intraocular inflammatory disease resistant to systemic corticosteroid and cytotoxic agents. *American Journal of Ophthalmology,* **96**, 275–282

NUSSENBLATT, R.B., PALESTINE, A.G., ROOK, A.H. *et al.* (1983) Treatment of intraocular inflammation with cyclosporin A. *Lancet,* **ii**, 235–238

O'DUFFY, J.D., ROBERTSON, D.M. and GOLDSTEIN, N.P. (1984) Chlorambucil in the treatment of uveitis and meningoencephalitis of Behçet's disease. *American Journal of Medicine,* **76**, 75–83

PALMER, R.G., KANSKI, J.J. and ANSELL, B.M. (1985) Chlorambucil in the treatment of intractable uveitis associated with juvenile chronic arthritis. *Journal of Rheumatology,* **12**, 967–970

11

Management of complicated cataract

Introduction

Cataract is a common complication of chronic anterior uveitis. The onset of cataract formation is characterized by a 'polychromatic lustre' at the posterior pole of the lens followed later by more extensive posterior (*Figure 11.1*) and anterior subcapsular opacification until the cataract becomes mature. The presence of extensive posterior synechiae may promote cataract formation and, in some cases, the prolonged use of systemic or topical steroids is also partly responsible.

Problems of management

The management of secondary cataracts due to uveitis frequently presents the surgeon with a considerable surgical challenge. This is because of the following, frequently inter-related, difficulties.

Diagnosis

The extent of lens opacities may be difficult to evaluate in eyes with band keratopathy (*Figure 11.2*) and small pupils due to extensive posterior synechiae. In some cases the anterior lens surface may also be covered by pigment or a fibrous membrane.

Timing of surgery

Although ideally, cataract surgery should be performed when the eye has been quiet for several weeks, this goal is frequently difficult to achieve because, in some patients, the intraocular inflammation responds poorly to medication and persists for many years. If in a young child surgery is delayed too long, an otherwise successful visual

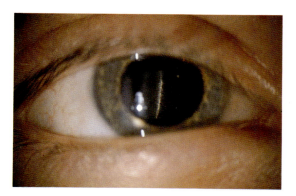

Figure 11.1 Early posterior cataract due to chronic anterior uveitis

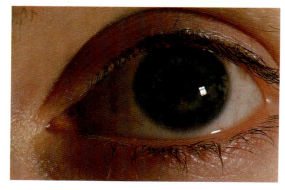

Figure 11.2 Band keratopathy and cataract

outcome may be compromised by irreversible stimulus-deprivation amblyopia.

Anaesthesia

In patients with arthritis intratracheal intubation may be difficult for the following reasons:
1 Neck extension may be restricted.

> *Note* Even patients with relatively mild peripheral arthritis may have severe involvement of the neck.

2 Movements of the jaw may be impaired by arthritis of the temporomandibular joints.
3 Failure of growth of the lower jaw in patients with juvenile chronic arthritis may interfere with visualization of the vocal cords, so that a 'blind' intubation through the nose may be necessary (*Figure 11.3*).

Intraocular inflammation

Since most eyes have active uveitis at the time of surgery, it is important to keep the amount of surgically induced exacerbation of intraocular inflammation to a minimum. This can be achieved by using procedures which inflict as little trauma as possible. Because a second operation should be avoided, other surgically treatable complications, such as band keratopathy and secondary glaucoma, should be corrected at the time of cataract surgery.

Post-operative pupillary membranes

An aphakic eye with active chronic anterior uveitis and an intact posterior capsule or an intact anterior hyaloid face is at risk of developing a secondary pupillary membrane (*Figure 11.4*). This is undesirable, not only because it impairs vision, but also because it requires further surgical intevention which, in turn, increases the amount of surgically induced uveitis and the risk of phthisis bulbi. The chosen technique should therefore have the capability of excising the anterior hyaloid face as well as the posterior capsule in order to eliminate the 'scaffold' along which membranes can develop.

Ocular hypotony

An eye with chronic anterior uveitis may have a low intraocular pressure due to hyposecretion of aqueous humour. This may be due to chronic inflammatory damage to the secretory ciliary epithelium or detachment of the ciliary body by a

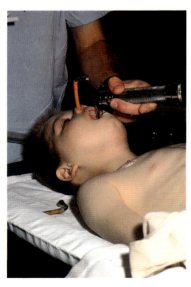

Figure 11.3 Intubation through nose

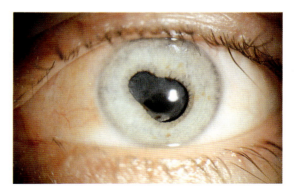

Figure 11.4 Opacification of anterior hyaloid face following cataract extraction

contracting cyclitic membrane. A hypotonous eye is susceptible to phthisis bulbi, particularly if subjected to severe and repeated surgical insults, e.g. needling of pupillary membranes.

Technical difficulties

Band keratopathy   If severe, this may impair visualization of the surgical field.

Ocular hypotony   This may make the surgical incision difficult.

Fibrous membrane   In eyes with long-standing uveitis, a fibrous membrane may cover the anterior lens surface (*Figure 11.5*).

Small pupil   Extensive posterior synechiae will interfere with access to the lens (*Figure 11.6*).

Rubeosis iridis   Some eyes with chronic uveitis develop neovascularization of the iris. In some cases, the blood vessels grow onto the anterior lens surface (*Figure 11.5*). Because these vessels do not possess the ability to contract when cut, they may be responsible for operative bleeding.

Shallow anterior chamber   Eyes with iris bombè have a shallow anterior chamber (*Figure 11.7*) making intraocular manipulation difficult.

Visual rehabilitation

Intraocular lenses   Due to the risk of secondary membrane formation in eyes with chronic anterior uveitis, intraocular lens implantation is contraindicated.

Soft contact lens   The continued need for topical steroid administration following cataract surgery in many patients, makes soft hydrophilic contact

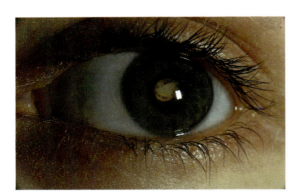

Figure 11.5 Fibrous membrane and blood vessels on anterior lens

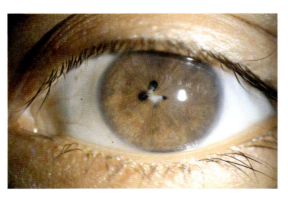

Figure 11.6 Extensive posterior synechiae and cataract

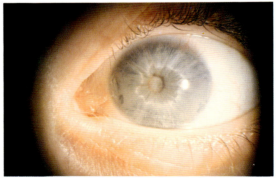

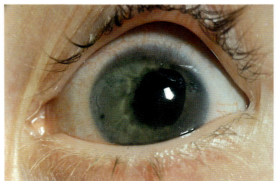

Figure 11.7 Top: iris bombè and cataract. Bottom: appearance following lensectomy

lenses inappropriate because the steroid will impregnate the lens.

Hard contact lens In most cases a hard daily wear contact lens which will not become impregnated is best.

Spectacles Bilateral aphakic patients who are unable to wear hard contact lenses can be fitted with spectacles.

Amblyopia

There is a danger that the surgeon may be so concerned with the technical success of cataract extraction that he forgets the possibility of amblyopia. Children with amblyopia should be referred to an orthoptist who is familiar with the problems of chronic intraocular inflammation and knows that failure of occlusion to improve visual acuity may be due to complications, such as pupillary membranes, band keratopathy, cystoid macular oedema and, occasionally, retinal detachment.

Surgical techniques

At present the three techniques used for cataract extraction are intracapsular, extracapsular and lensectomy.

Intracapsular extraction

Intracapsular surgery cannot be performed with safety in patients under the age of 35 years in whom the capsulo-hyaloidal ligament is still intact. If intracapsular surgery is attempted in young individuals, the risk of vitreous loss is unacceptably high. Although the enzyme alpha-chymotrypsin (Zonulysin) dissolves the zonule in a young person, it has no effect on the congenital adhesion between the anterior hyaloid face and the posterior capsule. In patients over the age of 35 years, intracapsular extraction is an acceptable procedure for cataracts secondary to uveitis. Eyes with small pupils from extensive posterior synechiae require a preliminary synechialysis and broad (sector) iridectomy prior to lens removal. If prolonged post-operative intraocular inflamma-

tion is anticipated, it is advisable to perform an anterior vitrectomy with a vitreous cutter in order to eliminate the anterior hyaloid face which can form a 'scaffold' for secondary membrane formation (*Figure 11.4*). The actual technique of intracapsular extraction is beyond the scope of this book.

Extracapsular extraction

Although extracapsular surgery is now a very popular method of treating uncomplicated senile cataracts, it is not an appropriate technique for removing cataracts secondary to anterior uveitis. This is because the posterior capsule and anterior vitreous remain intact and provide a 'scaffold' along which secondary membranes can proliferate post-operatively. Needling or YAG laser capsulotomy of the membranes does not eliminate this 'scaffold' and most of the openings in the capsule subsequently close and require further intervention. This repeated surgical insult to a severely compromised and chronically inflamed eye may set up a vicious circle—with exacerbation of uveitis, inflammatory damage to the secretory ciliary epithelium, hyposecretion of aqueous humour, and finally phthisis bulbi (*Figure 11.8*). Details of the technique of extracapsular extraction are beyond the scope of this book.

Lensectomy

This procedure involves the excision of the lens with an automated aspiration-cutting device (vit-

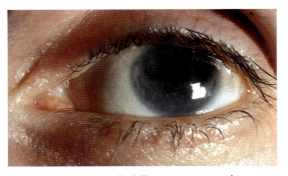

Figure 11.8 Phthisis bulbi following extracapsular cataract extraction

reous cutter) through a small limbal or pars plana incision. The technique is suitable only for soft cataracts in children and young adults because the lens material has to be soft enough to mould into the small aspiration port of the probe. Because many patients with cataracts secondary to uveitis are young, lensectomy can be used to treat a high proportion of cases. The main advantage of lensectomy is its ability to completely excise the posterior capsule, and a portion of the anterior vitreous. In this way the 'scaffold' for secondary membrane formation is eliminated.

In the past, a soft eye was considered a contraindication to surgical intervention for fear of precipitating phthisis. It now appears that, if lensectomy is carried out in a 'pre-phthisical' eye, the progressive downhill course to complete phthisis can be halted and even reversed. It is probably true to say that the presence of a low intraocular pressure in an eye with a cataract is an *indication* and not a contraindication to lensectomy. This is because some very soft eyes have a cyclitic membrane which is responsible for detachment of the ciliary body. If this membrane is excised at the time of lensectomy, the ciliary body becomes reattached and the secretory ciliary epithelium regains its normal function. Because lensectomy requires a very small incision, it can, if necessary, be combined with removal of band keratopathy or treatment of secondary glaucoma. However, it is important to point out that the operation is dependent on complex and expensive instrumentation. Ideally, the surgeon should be experienced in pars plana vitrectomy so that he has the necessary skill to retrieve lens fragments that may accidentally dislodge into the vitreous cavity. It should be remembered that, although with age the lens nucleus becomes harder, it is possible for a secondary cataract due to uveitis in a young child to be extremely hard and even calcified, so that the lens matter will not mould into the aspiration port of the cutter.

Preparation of patient for cataract surgery

The patient should be admitted two days prior to surgery and active intraocular inflammation treated with hourly or two-hourly dexamethasone drops. The routine use of systemic steroids during the peri-operative period is unnecessary. The pupil is dilated with atropine 1% drops instilled twice a day, if necessary supplemented with tropicamide 1% and phenylephrine 10% a few hours prior to surgery.

Instrumentation for lensectomy

The instruments necessary for lensectomy are a vitreous cutter (*Figure 11.9*), e.g. Ocutome, EMPAC, or SITE, a Graefe knife, Ziegler's knife, microforceps, microscissors (*Figure 11.10*), and intraocular cautery.

Incision for lensectomy

The operation can be performed through a limbal or a pars plana incision.

Advantages of limbal incision
1 Preferred by beginners as visualization of instruments is better.
2 In eyes with small pupils, sphincterotomy can be performed prior to lensectomy.
3 Complications associated with entry through the uvea (bleeding and uveal effusion) are avoided.

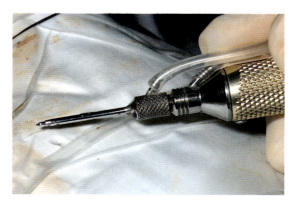

Figure 11.9 EMPAC vitreous cutter

Advantages of pars plana incision

1 A more complete excision is possible as access to lens material behind the iris is better.
2 The posterior segment can be visualized by placing a contact lens on the cornea. This is particularly useful in the event of accidental posterior dislocation of lens fragments during the operation. It also enables posterior vitrectomy to be performed in eyes with dense vitreous opacities.
3 There is less trauma to the iris and corneal endothelium.
4 The operation can be performed in the presence of a shallow anterior chamber.
5 The eye is more comfortable post-operatively.

Technique of lensectomy via pars plana

1 Check that the cutter is in good working order.
2 Insert a lid speculum and steady the globe with a superior rectus traction suture.

3 Make a small peritomy in the upper temporal quadrant (if you are right-handed and operating on the right eye) and extend with scissors to make a T-shaped incision (*Figure 11.11*).
4 Reflect conjunctiva and Tenon's capsule down to sclera (taking care not to damage the lateral rectus muscle).
5 With cautery make a mark on the sclera 3.5 mm behind the limbus.

> *Note* If you are not using a fully functioning probe (i.e. one with an infusion sleeve), repeat steps (3), (4) and (5) in the upper nasal quadrant and make a stab incision through sclera and uvea 3.5 mm from the limbus and secure the infusion cannula.

6 With a Graefe knife (or equivalent) make a stab incision through the sclera and uvea in the upper temporal quadrant 3.5 mm from the limbus (*Figure 11.12*).

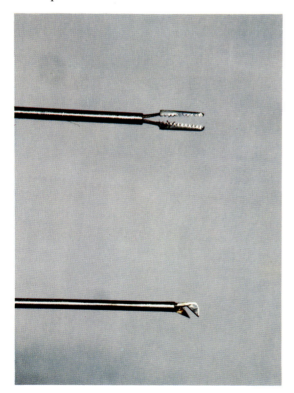

Figure 11.10 Top: microforceps; bottom: microscissors

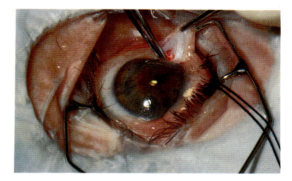

Figure 11.11 Conjunctival incision

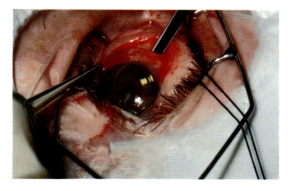

Figure 11.12 Scleral incision

7 Introduce the knife into the equator of the lens and then into the nucleus. Withdraw it slightly and puncture the anterior lens capsule (*Figure 11.13*).

8 Withdraw the Graefe knife from the eye and introduce a Ziegler's knife into the lens nucleus. Stir the lens matter, taking great care not to damage the posterior capsule. This manoeuvre facilitates the subsequent excision of the lens with the cutter.

Note If the knife does not enter the lens nucleus with ease or if it pushes the lens to the opposite side, this means that the nucleus is too hard to be aspirated into the cutting port. Do *not* proceed with lensectomy and consider one of two options: (*a*) suture the sclerotomy and convert to a large incision extracapsular extraction; (*b*) soften the lens nucleus with an ultrasonic fragmentor and then continue with the lensectomy.

---

9 Turn on the infusion system and introduce the tip of the cutter into the lens (*Figure 11.14*). If the sclerotomy is too small, enlarge it.

Note A tight fit is essential if leakage of fluid through the sclerotomy is to be avoided.

---

10 Remove the lens whilst working within the capsular bag. Relatively soft lens matter can be aspirated without activating the cutting mechanism, although harder pieces require both aspiration and cutting. Start with an aspiration pressure of 100 mmHg and, if necessary, increase it to 200 mmHg.

11 In order to visualize and excise peripheral lens matter from under the iris, indent the sclera and simultaneously rotate the globe towards the indented site. At all times, keep well away from the vitreous base.

Note In excising the peripheral cortical lens matter from under the iris, point the cutting port sideways. Pointing it upwards may aspirate iris, and pointing it posteriorly may cause premature damage to the posterior capsule with dislocation of lens material into the vitreous cavity.

---

12 Turn the cutting port posteriorly and excise the posterior capsule and anterior vitreous.

Note In eyes with severe and diffuse vitreous opacities, a total vitrectomy may be required.

---

13 Turn the cutting port anteriorly, engage the cut ends of the capsule, and excise it.

Note The anterior capsule is usually stronger than the posterior capsule.

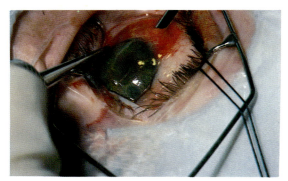

Figure 11.13 Puncture of anterior lens capsule

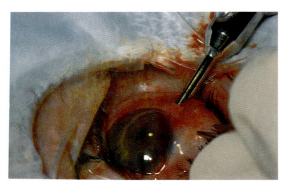

Figure 11.14 Insertion of cutter into lens

14 If the anterior lens capsule is covered by a dense rubbery fibrous plaque which cannot be excised, first cut free the plaque from surrounding tissue with vitreous microscissors (*Figure 11.15*), and then remove it with microforceps. Hard calcified plaques of lens matter that resist excision with the cutter can also be removed in this way.

15 Turn off the infusion system and aspirate a small amount of fluid through the cutter in order to lower the intraocular pressure. This will prevent herniation of intraocular contents through the sclerotomy when the cutter is withdrawn.

16 Gently withdraw the cutter from the eye and make sure that the sclerotomy is free from vitreous and uveal tissue.

17 Suture the sclerotomy with 6-0 Vicryl.

18 Suture the conjunctiva with 6-0 Vicryl or 6-0 catgut.

19 Give an anterior sub-Tenon injection of methylprednisolone (Depomedrone) and gentamicin (*Figure 11.16*).

Technique of lensectomy via limbus

1 If a fully functioning probe is not being used, insert a 25-gauge needle bevel down into the anterior chamber at the inferonasal limbus and attach it to an infusion system.

2 With a Graefe knife make a stab incision in peripheral clear cornea. Pass the knife through the centre of the pupil into the lens nucleus.

3 Introduce the tip of the cutter into the eye and, if necessary, enlarge the pupil (*Figure 11.17*).

4 Excise the lens whilst working within the capsular bag.

5 Excise the posterior capsule and perform an anterior vitrectomy.

6 Suture the incision with 10-0 nylon.

7 Give an anterior sub-Tenon injection of methylprednisolone and gentamicin.

The pre- and post-operative appearances of two cataracts treated by lensectomy are shown in *Figures 11.18* and *11.19*.

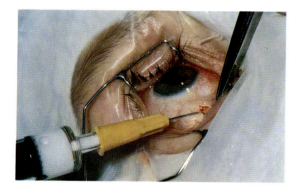

Figure 11.16 Anterior sub-Tenon injection

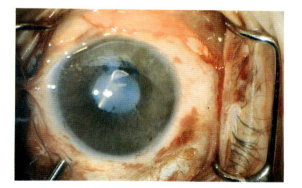

Figure 11.15 Cutting of tough plaque with microscissors

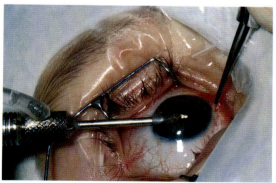

Figure 11.17 Enlargement of pupil with cutter

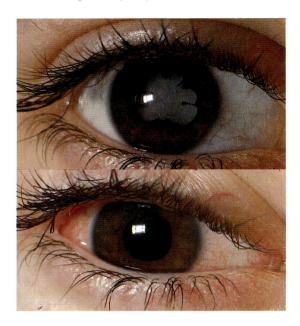

Figure 11.18 Top: pre-operative appearance; bottom: post-operative appearance

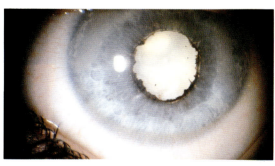

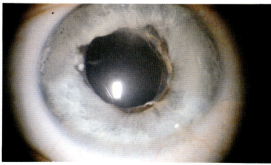

Figure 11.19 Top: pre-operative appearance; bottom: post-operative appearance

Complications of lensectomy

Accidental iridectomy This may occur if excessive suction pressure is used when working near the iris, or if the aspiration port is pointing upwards when under the iris. If iris tissue is accidentally aspirated (*Figure 11.20*) use the reflex capability (if available) to disengage.

Posterior dislocation of lens material This is caused by:

1 Premature damage to the posterior capsule with the Graefe knife during the initial incision.
2 Premature damage to the posterior capsule with the cutter during lens excision.
3 Attempted excision of a hard nucleus.

Management Small lens fragments can be left alone but large pieces, especially if composed of hard nucleus, must be removed as they frequently float into the anterior chamber post-operatively where they may damage the corneal endothelium.

Technique of extraction of soft fragments (Figure 11.21 left)
1 Place a contact lens on the cornea.

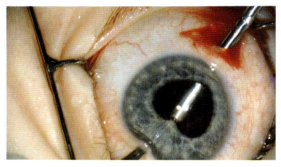

Figure 11.20 Accidental aspiration of iris into cutting port

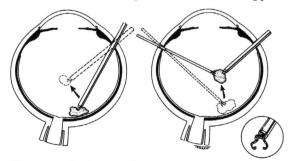

Figure 11.21 Technique of extraction of dislodged lens fragments. Left: for soft fragments; right: for hard fragments

2 Apply the tip of the cutter with the aspiration port open to the lens fragment—taking great care not to touch the retina. Apply gentle suction until the fragment is impacted. Slowly retract the probe into the midvitreous cavity, apply strong suction and excise the fragment by activating the cutting mode.

Technique of extraction of hard fragments (Figure 11.21 right)

1 Make a pars plana incision in the upper nasal quadrant (if the cutter is positioned in the upper temporal quadrant) and place a contact lens on the cornea.

2 Introduce microforceps through the nasal sclerotomy and pick up the lens fragments. With the forceps and the cutter in the midvitreous cavity, feed the lens particle into the aspiration port and excise. Repeat several times until all fragments have been removed.

Note It is also possible to crush the lens fragments between the tip of the cutter and the fibreoptic light pipe. Each small particle can then be excised with the cutter.

Bleeding Intra-operative haemorrhage can usually be controlled by elevating the intraocular pressure. Persistent bleeding points can be cauterized directly (*Figure 11.22*).

Retinal dialysis This extremely serious complication is due to traction on the peripheral retina by aspiration of solid vitreous in the region of the vitreous base—keep well away from the vitreous base, examine the retina routinely after the completion of lensectomy and repair a dialysis immediately by cryotherapy and plombage.

Further reading

DANGEL, M.E., STARK, W.J. and MICHELS, R.G. (1983) Surgical management of cataract associated with chronic uveitis. *Ophthalmic Surgery*, **14**, 145–149

DIAMOND, J.G. and KAPLAN, H.J. (1978) Lensectomy and vitrectomy for complicated cataract secondary to uveitis. *Archives of Ophthalmology*, **96**, 1798–1804

FISHER, R.F. (1981) The lens in uveitis. *Transactions of the Ophthalmological Society of the United Kingdom*, **101**, 317–320

KANSKI, J.J. and CRICK, M.D.P. (1977) Lensectomy. *Transactions of the Ophthalmological Society of the United Kingdom*, **97**, 52–57

NOLTHENIUS, P.A.T. and DEUTMAN, A.F. (1983) Surgical treatment of the complications of chronic uveitis. *Ophthalmologica*, **186**, 11–16

PRAEGER, D.L., SCHNEIDER, H.A., SAKOWSKI, A.D. *et al.* (1976) Kelman procedure in the treatment of complicated cataract of the uveitis of Still's disease. *Transactions of the Ophthalmological Society of the United Kingdom*, **96**, 168–171

REYNARD, M. and MINCKNER, D.S. (1983) Cataract extraction in the sympathizing eye. *Archives of Ophthalmology*, **101**, 1701–1703

SMITH, R.E. and O'CONNOR, G.R. (1974) Cataract extraction in Fuchs' syndrome. *Archives of Ophthalmology*, **91**, 39–41

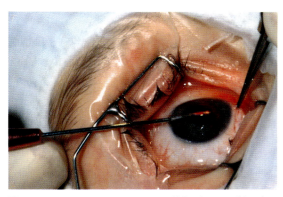

Figure 11.22 Direct cauterization of bleeding iris blood vessels

12

Management of secondary glaucoma

Introduction

Secondary inflammatory glaucoma frequently presents the clinician with a considerable diagnostic and therapeutic challenge. Although in some cases the elevation of intraocular pressure (IOP) is transient and innocuous, frequently it is persistent and severely damaging. In fact, secondary glaucoma is now the most common cause of blindness in eyes with chronic anterior uveitis, particularly in children.

Diagnostic problems

Failure to monitor IOP

The clinician may be so preoccupied with suppressing the intraocular inflammation, that he may fail to suspect the presence of raised IOP. He may also have the mistaken belief that a young and healthy optic disc can withstand prolonged periods of raised IOP and remain unscathed.

High swings in IOP

The diurnal fluctuation of IOP, normally exaggerated in eyes with primary open-angle glaucoma, are even more dramatic in eyes with a compromised outflow facility due to chronic anterior uveitis. It is therefore important to monitor patients with borderline pressures over a 24-h period (phasing).

Ciliary shutdown

Acute iridocyclitis or an acute exacerbation of chronic iridocyclitis is frequently associated with a temporary decrease in aqueous secretion due to inflammation of the secretory ciliary epithelium (ciliary shutdown). The finding of a normal or subnormal IOP may therefore lull the clinician into a false sense of security, so that he may overlook the fact that a return of ciliary body function, due to a decrease in uveitis activity, may be associated with a rise in IOP in an eye with a permanently compromised outflow facility. It is therefore important to perform gonioscopy on all eyes with chronic anterior uveitis and to continue to monitor the IOP and the appearance of the optic discs as the inflammation is resolving.

Mechanism

In some cases it may be difficult to determine the actual mechanism of the pressure rise and, in some cases, more than one mechanism may be responsible. In steroid responders, the IOP may become elevated as the inflammation is being brought under control.

Classification

Secondary glaucoma due to anterior uveitis can be divided into four main types. As already mentioned more than one mechanism may play a part in the same eye.

1 Angle-closure due to pupil block.
2 Angle-closure without pupil block.
3 Open-angle.
4 Specific hypertensive uveitis syndromes.

Angle-closure from pupil block

Mechanism

Secondary angle-closure is caused by 360° iridolenticular adhesions (seclusio pupillae). Since the pupil block obstructs the passage of aqueous humour from the posterior to the anterior chamber, the increased pressure in the posterior chamber causes an anterior bowing of the peripheral iris (iris bombè). Severe iris bombè is associated with shallowing of the anterior chamber and apposition of the peripheral iris to the trabeculum and peripheral cornea. If the eye has active inflammation, the iridocorneal contact soon becomes permanent with the development of peripheral anterior synechiae (PAS).

Very occasionally, pupil block develops in an aphakic eye due to adhesion between the iris sphincter and an organized anterior vitreous face or an intact posterior capsule. This is one of the reasons for avoiding extracapsular cataract extraction in eyes with chronic anterior uveitis and performing an anterior vitrectomy following intracapsular cataract surgery.

Diagnosis

Secondary angle-closure glaucoma due to seclusio pupillae is now relatively rare. In fact, most eyes with seclusio pupillae have a normal or a subnormal IOP due to concomitant chronic ciliary shutdown or detachment of the ciliary body by a contracting cyclitic membrane.

Slitlamp biomicroscopy shows 360° posterior synechiae, iris bombè, and a shallow anterior chamber. Gonioscopy shows apposition of the peripheral iris to the trabeculum and, in advanced cases, also to the peripheral cornea. Indentation gonioscopy with a Zeiss four-mirror goniolens may be useful in assessing the extent of angle closure by reversible (appositional) contact and how much is closed by permanent PAS. The central part of the cornea is indented by pressing the goniolens posteriorly. This displaces the aqueous humour into the periphery of the anterior chamber and tends to separate the peripheral iris from the angle structures. In the absence of

permanent PAS, the peripheral iris will be pushed back and the trabeculum visualized. In eyes with permanent PAS the iris will remain adherent to the trabeculum.

Note Indentation gonioscopy is of no value in eyes with very high IOPs.

Medical management

Prevention of seclusio pupillae

In the majority of cases, seclusio pupillae can be prevented by adequate therapy. In eyes with acute anterior uveitis, atropine should be used to prevent posterior synechiae, whereas in eyes with chronic anterior uveitis, a short-acting mydriatic such as tropicamide 1% or cyclopentolate 1%, instilled once or twice a day, is effective in preventing formation of posterior synechiae by keeping the pupil mobile. Once significant posterior synechiae have formed, topical mydriatics (atropine, phenylephrine, cocaine) are seldom effective in breaking them down although an anterior sub-Tenon injection of Mydricaine (a mixture of atropine, adrenaline, and procaine) may be effective if the synechiae are relatively new and unassociated with fibrosis.

Prevention of PAS

In an eye with active anterior uveitis, PAS will form quickly once the peripheral iris is apposed to the trabeculum. In the presence of appositional angle closure, it is therefore extremely important to reduce the 'stickiness' of the peripheral iris as quickly as possible with intensive topical steroids and an anterior sub-Tenon injection of methylprednisolone acetate (Depomedrone).

Lowering of IOP

Although some eyes with healthy optic discs are able to tolerate a moderately high IOP for several weeks, it is important to reduce the IOP as soon as possible, particularly if surgery is being contemplated. In relatively mild cases, topical therapy with timolol, adrenaline and propine may be effective, although when the pressure is very high carbonic anhydrase inhibitors (acetazolamide, dichlorphenamide) are usually also required. However, it is important to point out that hyperosmotic agents (mannitol, glycerol), whose action is dependent on an intact blood–aqueous barrier may be less effective in lowering IOP than in eyes with primary angle-closure glaucoma.

Surgical management

Laser iridotomy

If medical therapy is ineffective, the communication between the posterior and anterior chambers should be re-established without delay by performing an iridotomy or iridectomy. However, this will be successful only if less than 75% of the angle is permanently closed with PAS. In eyes with relatively thick irides, a YAG laser may be more effective than an argon laser in penetrating the iris stroma. In eyes with shallow anterior chambers, great care should be taken not to damage the corneal endothelium. Although laser iridotomy is safer than surgical iridectomy in eyes with intraocular inflammation, it has the disadvantage that the opening in the iris is smaller (particularly with the YAG laser) and more prone to subsequent closure in eyes with persistent inflammation. For this reason, it is recommended that several iridotomies are performed and the patient is examined at frequent intervals to ensure that the openings remain patent.

Surgical iridectomy

This should be considered only if laser iridotomy is unsuccessful or if a laser is unavailable. Pre-operatively every effort should be made to reduce the amount of intraocular inflammation as much as possible and to lower the IOP medically. An incision should be made in clear cornea and care should be taken to avoid a rapid decompression of the globe. In order to lessen the possibility of post-operative closure, a sector (broad) rather than a peripheral iridectomy should be performed. The anterior chamber should be reconstituted with great care, because a shallow anterior chamber will

predispose to PAS formation and negate the effects of the operation.

> *Note*   Since it is not always possible to determine the extent of permanent angle-closure by PAS, it is recommended that, if medical treatment fails, all eyes are treated by laser iridotomy or surgical iridectomy. The management of eyes unresponsive to these measures is similar to that of secondary angle-closure glaucoma unassociated with pupil block (*see* later).

Angle-closure without pupil block

Mechanism

In phakic eyes

In eyes with chronic iridocyclitis, the deposition and subsequent contraction of inflammatory debris may pull the peripheral iris over the trabeculum and cause a gradual and progressive closure of the angle by PAS. Eyes with pre-existing narrow angles are more at risk from angle-closure than those with open angles. Eyes with granulomatous inflammation (*see Figure 12.1*) may also be

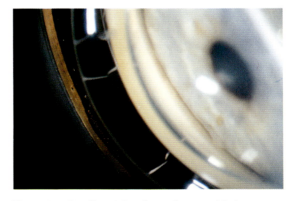

Figure 12.1 Small peripheral anterior synechia in eye with granulomatous anterior uveitis (courtesy of Mr M. Sanders)

more prone to this type of angle-closure than those with non-granulomatous uveitis.

In aphakic eyes

Secondary glaucoma is a relatively common complication following surgery for complicated cataracts. It has been postulated that this may be due in part to failure to reconstitute the anterior chamber immediately after the completion of surgery. Air should be avoided as it may predispose to PAS formation and the anterior chamber should be reconstituted with either saline or balanced salt solution. In addition, inadequate post-operative suppression of surgically induced inflammation may promote the formation of PAS.

Diagnosis

Secondary angle-closure unassociated with pupil block is a common cause of raised IOP in eyes with chronic iridocyclitis. As the angle becomes progressively compromised, the rise in IOP is usually gradual. Even severe elevations of IOP of 50 mmHg or more may be asymptomatic or the patient may merely report an occasional mild headache. Because of this relative lack of symptoms and a slitlamp examination which merely shows a deep anterior chamber, it is extremely important to constantly monitor the IOP, examine the angle gonioscopically, and evaluate the optic discs for evidence of glaucomatous damage. In very young and uncooperative children, tonometry and gonioscopy may be extremely difficult or impossible and the first suspicion of glaucoma is the finding of a grossly cupped optic disc. As already mentioned, exacerbations of intraocular inflammation in eyes with chronic iridocyclitis are frequently associated with a lowering of IOP. Even glaucomatous eyes with a moderate elevation of IOP of 30–35 mmHg may become hypotonous during acute exacerbations. It is therefore extremely important to pay particular attention to the IOP as the uveitis is being brought under control.

Management

The problems encountered in the management of inflammatory glaucoma due to angle-closure by extensive PAS are surpassed only by that of treatment of neovascular glaucoma. In fact, some eyes with inflammatory glaucoma develop a fibrovascular membrane in the angle, similar to that seen in neovascular glaucoma. The following options should be considered.

Non-intervention

In eyes with relatively mild iridocyclitis, it may be prudent not to treat the inflammation too vigorously for fear of upsetting the delicate balance between diminished aqueous outflow and decreased inflow as a result of relative ciliary body shutdown.

Medical

Topical therapy with timolol, adrenaline and propine may be effective in mild cases, although moderate to severe cases require the addition of carbonic anhydrase inhibitors to bring the IOP down to a safe level.

> *Note* Miotics should not be used as they promote the formation of posterior synechiae and also exacerbate the intraocular inflammation.

Filtration surgery

This may be successful in some adult eyes, but the results are inferior to those in primary open-angle glaucoma. The results of filtration surgery are particularly disappointing in children. Some of the possible reasons are: (1) a low scleral rigidity in children predisposes to complications such as vitreous loss, scleral collapse, and scleral ectasia, and (2) the increased thickness and more rapid healing of Tenon's capsule predisposes to obstruction of the sclerotomy site.

Trabeculodialysis

This procedure is performed with an irrigating goniotomy needle (*Figure 12.2*). The tip of the needle is passed across the anterior chamber into the inferior angle and PAS are retracted by depressing the base of the iris (*Figure 12.3*). An incision is then made just posterior to Schwalbe's line and the trabeculum is retracted. If possible, the incision should be extended for about 90°. It has been postulated that the mechanism by which trabeculodialysis lowers IOP is by providing a direct communication between the anterior chamber and Schlemm's canal. The main advantages of this procedure are: (1) it is relatively easy to perform, (2) it is free from serious complications, and (3) it can be combined with lensectomy. Trabeculodialysis is successful in lowering IOP in about 60% of eyes with severe inflammatory glaucoma although may patients still need medical therapy. Interestingly, the presence of aphakia and the extent of pre-operative angle closure have no bearing on the surgical outcome.

Goniosynechialysis

This relatively new procedure involves first deepening of the anterior chamber with sodium hyaluronate (Healonid) followed by separation of the PAS under direct visualization with a special curved irrigating cyclodialysis spatula. This operation may be successful provided the angle has not been closed for longer than one year.

Valve implants (Figure 12.4)

In some eyes, valve implants (Molteno, White, Schocket) may be successful in lowering IOP.

Cyclocryotherapy (Figure 12.5)

This procedure consists of destruction of the secretory ciliary epithelium. A special glaucoma probe or a retinal cryoprobe is used with the applications placed 3 mm from the limbus with freezing at −80 °C for one minute. Initially 180° of the globe should be treated with six applications. When re-treatment is required the same area

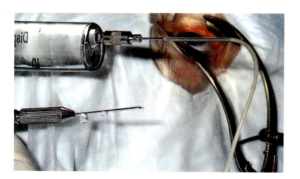

Figure 12.2 Irrigating goniotomy needle used for trabeculodialysis

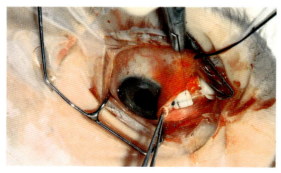

Figure 12.4 Insertion of 'White' valve implant

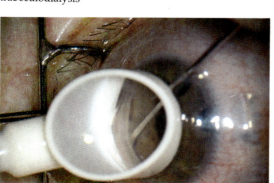

Figure 12.3 Retraction of peripheral anterior synechiae with tip of goniotomy needle

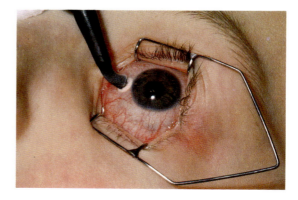

Figure 12.5 Cyclocryotherapy

should be frozen and only if this is ineffective should the remaining 180° of the globe be treated in a similar fashion. The main disadvantages of this procedure are the risk of inducing phthisis bulbi and that, in many cases, the IOP drop is only temporary.

Open-angle glaucoma

Mechanism

In acute iridocyclitis

As already mentioned during the acute phase of anterior uveitis, the IOP is usually normal or subnormal due to a concomitant ciliary shutdown. Occasionally, however, a secondary open-angle glaucoma develops due to obstruction of aqueous outflow, most commonly just as the acute inflammation is subsiding and ciliary body function is returning to normal. This effect, which is transient and fairly innocuous, may be steroid induced or caused by a combination of the following mechanisms.

Trabecular obstruction Inflammatory cells and debris may clog the intertrabecular pores and the trabecular obstruction may be associated with increased aqueous viscosity due to leakage of proteins from the inflamed iris blood vessels. Eventually the cells and debris are phagocytosed by the trabecular endothelial cells and, provided the uveitis does not recur, the trabeculum regains its full facility of outflow and the IOP returns to normal.

Acute trabeculitis A reduction in outflow facility may be caused by inflammation and oedema of the trabeculum itself, with a secondary reduction in the diameter of the trabecular pores. It is thought that acute trabeculitis is the probable cause of raised IOP in eyes with uveitis due to herpes zoster and herpes simplex.

Prostaglandins These may be associated with raised IOP although the exact mechanisms are still uncertain.

In chronic iridocyclitis

It has been postulated that the main mechanism for reduced outflow facility in eyes with open angles and chronic anterior uveitis is trabecular scarring and/or sclerosis as a result of chronic trabeculitis. The exact incidence and importance of this mechanism is, however, difficult to determine with accuracy as most eyes also have PAS.

Diagnosis

Due to the variable appearance of the chamber angle on gonioscopy, a definitive diagnosis of elevated IOP as a result of reduced facility of outflow is very difficult. In theory, the angle should be open and in some eyes a gelatinous exudate resembling 'mashed potatoes' may be seen on the trabeculum.

Management

In acute iridocyclitis, the IOP usually returns to normal once the inflammation has subsided. In steroid-responders, it may be necessary to discontinue strong steroids (dexamethasone, betamethasone) and use a weaker steroid such as fluorometholone which has a lower propensity for elevating IOP. In chronic iridocyclitis the treatment is similar to that of secondary angle-closure glaucoma by PAS.

Specific hypertensive uveitis syndromes

Fuchs' uveitis syndrome

See Chapter 8.

Glaucomatocyclitic crisis (Posner–Schlossman syndrome)

See Chapter 9.

Further reading

CAMPBELL, D.G. and VELA, A. (1984) Modern gonio-synechialysis for the treatment of synechial angle-closure glaucoma. *Ophthalmology*, **91**, 1052–1060

CAPRIOLI, J., STRANG, S.L. and SPAETH, G.L. (1985) Cyclocryotherapy in the treatment of advanced glaucoma. *Ophthalmology*, **92**, 947–954

HERSCHLER, J. and DAVIS, E.B. (1980) Modified goniotomy for inflammatory glaucoma; histologic evidence for the mechanism of pressure reduction. *Archives of Ophthalmology*, **98**, 684–687

HOSKINS, H.D. JR, HETHERINGTON, J. JR and SHAFFER, R.N. (1977) Surgical management of inflammatory glaucoma. *Perspectives in Ophthalmology*, **1**, 173–181

KANSKI, J.J. and McALLISTER, J.A. (1985) Trabeculodialysis for inflammatory glaucoma in children and young adults. *Ophthalmology*, **92**, 927–929

RITCH, R. (1981) Pathophysiology of glaucoma in uveitis. *Transactions of the Ophthalmological Society of the United Kingdom*, **101**, 321–324

SARKIES, N.J.C. and HITCHINGS, R.A. (1985) Silicone tube and gutter in advanced glaucoma. *Transactions of the Ophthalmological Society of the United Kingdom*, **104**, 133–136

SCHOCKET, S.S., NIRANKARI, V.S., LAKHANPAL, V. *et al.* (1985) Anterior chamber tube shunt to an encircling band in the treatment of neovascular glaucoma and other refractory glaucomas. *Ophthalmology*, **92**, 553–562

Index